DOWNLOAD YOUR FREE
QUICKSTART GUIDE

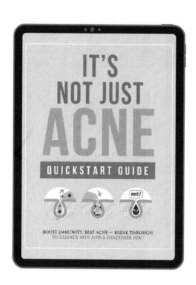

www.DrShaynaPeter.com/Quickstart

Purchase The Audiobook at:

www.DrShaynaPeter.com/audio

Do You Want A Personalized Wellness Program Tailored to You?

Do You Want A Proven Step-by-Step System to Follow?

If you answered yes to either of these questions, visit the link below to learn more about our programs and schedule a call with our team.

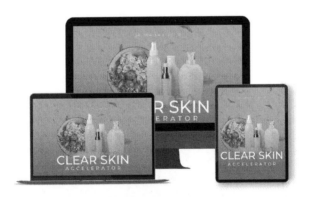

Schedule A Call At:

WellAheadChicago.com/call

IT'S
NOT JUST
ACNE

IT'S NOT JUST ACNE

BOOST IMMUNITY, BEAT ACNE — BREAK THROUGH
TO CLEARER SKIN AND A HEALTHIER YOU!

DR. SHAYNA E. PETER

Disclaimer: This publication contains the book opinions and ideas of the author based on their education, experience, and research. The information contained within this publication is intended to help the reader make informed decisions about their health and is not to be construed as medical advice or treatment. All readers should consult with their health care provider before adopting any suggestions given in this publication, making any changes to their medical treatment plan. If you suspect you have a medical problem, we encourage you to seek competent medical help.

ISBN 978-1-7354657-0-8 paperback

ISBN 978-1-7354657-3-9 hardcover

ISBN 978-1-7354657-1-5 ebook

ISBN 978-1-7354657-2-2 audiobook

Distributed by Ingram Spark

Cover design by Haresh Makwana

Layout design by G Sharp Design, LLC.

DEDICATION

This book is dedicated to my patients and clients. I have learned so much from you! Thank you for giving me the opportunity to be part of your health journey and for being an absolute pleasure to work with.

TABLE OF CONTENTS

INTRODUCTION

If you are tired of struggling with acne and are looking for answers, this book is for you. If you have tried a lot of the standard treatments for acne without much success or if you have been dealing with severe acne and want treatment options other than harsh medications that come with dangerous side effects, this book is for you. This book is for you if you recognize that persistent acne is not just a skin problem but a signal of a more serious issue and you want to dig deeper. Perhaps acne is just one of many symptoms you are dealing with, and you have a feeling that your other symptoms could be related. You want to achieve full-body wellness! You're frustrated and tired of trying everything under the sun to get rid of your acne.

This book gives an introduction to the approach that we use to address acne in my functional medicine practice. I've designed the content to help you get past limiting beliefs when it comes to acne and to truly understand the potential root causes behind this complex skin condition.

STRUCTURE OF THIS BOOK

I designed this book to guide you through understanding and identifying the root causes behind acne step-by-step. I also want to help you understand what other symptoms you might be experiencing that could be related to acne and how balancing your immune system is the key to achieving long-term relief. We will also talk about what habit and lifestyle changes you can make in order to promote clear skin. We are going to get you on the path to recovery!

CHAPTER ONE

THE STRUGGLE IS REAL

If you've been dealing with acne for a while, you might feel ready to throw in the towel, but I want to assure you that there is hope. First, you need to reframe how you are viewing this whole situation. I know that acne can be quite a nuisance, but what you have is not a burden—it's a gift and an opportunity. I know it may not seem like a gift right now, but when you think about it, would you rather have your health fall apart all of a sudden, or would you rather have a warning sign you can act on? Throughout these pages, I will share stories of people just like you who have gone from having severe acne to having clear skin. My goal is to take you from an acne sufferer to an acne conqueror!

The first step toward recovery is letting go of the frustration about treatments that have not worked in the past. If you are reading this book, chances are you might feel like you've tried literally a million different skin care products, facials, aesthetic procedures, doctor's appointments, different types of diets, supplements...and yet you still have acne and you are still on an endless hamster wheel. You may have even spent a lot of money on all of these different treatments. Sometimes the most frustrating part is that you *did start to see results, but* then the acne eventually came back. That's when you knew the root cause had not been addressed.

QUALITY OF LIFE

Acne can be a very stubborn and distressing condition—just ask anyone who's struggled with it! What you thought was supposed to be a teenage struggle has followed you into adulthood.

Having severe acne may also have made you feel isolated. What has acne prevented you from doing in your life? Maybe you don't have the confidence to date or leave the house without makeup. Maybe you've become an introvert and a homebody as a result of acne. Think about how having clear skin will change your life! It could be something as simple as spending less time getting ready in the morning because you won't have to put on a lot of makeup before leaving the house in order to feel comfortable in public. You also won't have to spend so much money on makeup to cover things up—instead, you'll have a natural glow to your skin.

Or will the change be even deeper? Will having clear skin thrust your confidence to a whole different level, one where you're able to feel comfortable in your own skin and be more social? Maybe acne has been causing you to withdraw socially and fade into the background, or maybe it has been preventing you from having the type of social life and relationships you want. Has it been preventing you from dating? Have you not been able fully appreciate your naturally given beauty because your skin is covered with acne?

If acne is one of the ways your body alerts you to an imbalance, it's not exactly realistic to think that if you use the right skin care product or treat the root causes, you will never have another breakout. However, can you see a dramatic improvement? Absolutely. Can you get to the point where your skin is clear most of the time? Absolutely. Once you've addressed the root causes, it's about maintenance.

Even though acne can be depressing, disfiguring, and frankly annoying, the best thing you can do for yourself right now is change how you're looking at it. What you actually have is an opportunity to optimize your health by listening to your skin and listening to your body. We have to shift our mindset from thinking that the same treatment will work for everyone with the same condition. On the contrary, treatment approaches to acne sometimes have to be as individual as the person.

The first step in getting to the bottom of acne is realizing that **acne is an external expression of an internal imbalance.** This can be caused by a variety of factors that have to be addressed and kept in balance in order to achieve and maintain clear skin.

Addressing the various factors discussed in this book can keep breakouts at bay. A holistic approach can improve acne *and* have the side effect of improved overall health.

On your journey toward clear skin, it's important to give acne a positive spin. A visible alarm that something is off can be better than an *invisible alarm. If you listen, you'll have the opportunity to experience better health than you ever thought possible. Above all,* as you journey toward clear skin, chase health, not perfection.

MY STORY

Here's something a lot of people may not know about me. What I'm about to share changed the course of my health, my career, and ultimately my life. It's also a big reason why I'm committed to helping people understand the root causes behind skin problems.

When I was in medical school on the path to becoming a dermatologist, I started to struggle with acne for the first time in my life. I tried nearly every medication, skin product, facial, and cosmetic treatment out there, and I had the experience of conventional treatment methods failing me as a patient. Most of the treatments irritated my skin, made it very dry, and did not give me any lasting relief. Underneath it all, I knew there had to be a deeper root cause that was being ignored.

Meanwhile, as a medical student gaining exposure in dermatology, I saw many patients with severe acne. I saw a lot of the concerns and reservations they had about some of the standard treatments for acne, whether that was antibiotics, Accutane, birth control, or other hormone-regulating medications. Many parents were especially concerned about starting their teenage children on these treatments. I saw all of the counseling and consent forms that had to be signed and all of the precautionary protocols that had to be followed in order for patients to be able to start Accutane because of its high potential for adverse effects.

As a doctor in training, I wanted to be able to truly "do no harm" and offer my future patients safer treatment options that would address the root causes of their concerns. These experiences are what led me to functional medicine as first a patient and then a practitioner. These same experiences continue to fuel my passion about and commitment to helping people with skin conditions and autoimmune disorders.

Being prone to acne myself became a gift. It has given me insight into my health that I wouldn't have had otherwise. I honestly think that my health would be worse if struggling with acne had not forced me to dig deeper into my health issues.

CHAPTER TWO

IT'S NOT JUST ACNE

We've been conditioned over the years to think of acne as a cosmetic thing, a vanity issue. However, it's actually on the autoimmune spectrum. What this means is that acne can be one of the first signs of an autoimmune process brewing. If the root causes are not identified and addressed, the same triggers that cause acne can progress to a full blown autoimmune condition over time. If you've been struggling with acne, it's really important to understand the gravity of the condition and take it seriously. I'm not saying to obsess over every pimple, but if your acne has been a chronic issue, you need to recognize that there's an internal problem. Here are some examples of internal issues that have been linked to acne in medical research:

➤ Cystic acne is associated with an increased risk of prostate cancer and breast cancer

➤ Chronic inflammation from acne is associated with higher incidence of melanoma

- → Irritable bowel syndrome (IBS)
- → Insulin resistance
- → Small intestinal bacterial overgrowth (SIBO)
- → Autoimmune issues
- → Depression (in many cases, acne and depression can be a forward-feeding cycle, because derangements in the gut microbiome not only cause acne, they also alter neurotransmitter balance; to make matters worse, the psychological effects of acne can also fuel depression)
- → Anxiety
- → Hidradenitis suppurativa
- → Respiratory infections
- → Overweight/obesity

If you have other symptoms—constipation, loose stools, stomach cramps, recurrent yeast infections, urinary tract infections, stubborn weight gain, headaches, brain fog, fatigue—I'm here to tell you that even though you may have gotten used to living this way, it's not normal. These symptoms are common, yes, but they're not normal. And there could very well be a correlation between your symptoms and your acne. As you pinpoint the root causes behind your acne and do the work to correct those imbalances, you will likely see an improvement in your other symptoms as well.

HOW TO HEAL ACNE FROM THE INSIDE OUT

Get inflammation under control—while acne is not a full-blown autoimmune condition, it is on the autoimmune spectrum and can be one of the first signs of the beginning stages of an autoimmune dysfunction. It's good to keep in mind that auto-immune disorders don't develop overnight—for most people, it takes decades. It's a wise move to pay attention to early signals like acne. Throughout this book, we'll cover how to:

- ➜ Optimize vitamin and mineral levels
- ➜ Balance hormones
- ➜ Avoid inflammatory foods
- ➜ Optimize digestive function
- ➜ Correct dysbiosis
- ➜ Heal leaky gut
- ➜ Support detoxification
- ➜ Reduce skin inflammation

CHAPTER THREE

NUTRITIONAL DEFICIENCIES

"The doctor of the future will give no medicine but will interest their patients in the care of the human frame, in diet, and in the cause and prevention of disease."

~THOMAS EDISON

➙ Do you have low energy levels?

➙ Do you consume alcohol regularly?

➙ Do you regularly take prescription or over-the-counter medications?

➙ Have you been pregnant in the last two years?

➙ Have you had more than one pregnancy within a two-year period?

➙ Do you do strength training regularly?

➙ Do you have a diagnosed autoimmune condition?

➙ Are you following a special diet (i.e., vegan, gluten-free, keto)?

➙ Do you feel fullness one to three hours after eating?

We are accustomed to thinking of health in terms of the number of calories we consume or perhaps what gives us energy and what does not. We are led by our cravings and one question: "Does it taste good?" Our fast-paced lives only exacerbate this perception, causing us to live to eat rather than to eat so that we can live.

When we are hungry, it is a signal that we need nutrients, not just calories. If we take it upon ourselves to understand nutrition, we advance towards self-maintenance and healing in general. Specifically, in the case of acne, key nutrients can work to reduce inflammation, stabilize hormones, and repair damage to your skin cells, thus healing scar tissue. When you allow your diet to work as your medicine, you are literally creating the opportunity to heal your skin twenty-four hours a day. Optimal nutrition works around the clock!

NUTRITIONAL DEFICIENCIES

Many vitamins and minerals affect acne either directly or indirectly. In this chapter, we're going to cover some of the most common nutritional deficiencies of acne sufferers. This is not an exhaustive list, but it does cover the vitamins and minerals (and their associated functions) that are most relevant to acne. It's also important to remember that *all* nutrients work together.

OMEGA-3, OMEGA-6, AND OMEGA-9 FATTY ACIDS

There are three categories of essential fatty acids: omega-3, omega-6, and omega-9. A proper balance of these essential fatty acids is needed in order to help to maintain our cell membranes. In standard American diets, there is usually an excess of omega-6, and this excess promotes inflammation. Omega-3 fatty acids, in contrast, are anti-inflammatory. Maintaining an optimal ratio of omega-3 to omega-6 helps control the levels of inflammation in the body. Eicosapentaenoic acid (EPA) and Docosahexaenoic acid (DHA) are examples of omega-3 fatty acids that are isolated and used in some supplemental formulas.

There's a specific ratio you should know about, and that's your arachidonic acid to EPA ratio. This ratio is a marker for inflammation within your cells. (Arachidonic acid is an omega-6 fatty acid.) Having a balanced ratio of arachidonic acid to EPA helps keep the sebum produced in our sebaceous glands from becoming too thick and sticky. When the sebum does become sticky, it's more likely to clog pores in the skin and create acne.

Omega-3 fatty acids also facilitate mental health, weight reduction, and the reduction of liver fat. The chemical structure of omega-6 is slightly different from omega-3, although both are polyunsaturated fats. Omega-6 fatty acids are primarily used for energy. The most common one is linoleic acid. Both omega-3 and omega-6 fatty acids are polyunsaturated fats, and because our bodies cannot produce them, we need to consume them. (Although again, most Americans consume too many omega-6 fatty acids.)

Omega-9 fatty acids are the third type of omega fatty acids, and they are monounsaturated fats. In contrast to omega-3 and omega-6 fatty acids, our bodies can manufacture small amounts of omega-9 fatty acids. Omega-9 fatty acids reduce inflammation, decrease insulin resistance, and increase metabolism. The key to getting the health benefits of omega fatty acids is maintaining the proper balance of omega-3, omega-6, and omega-9.

In addition to omega-3 and omega-6, omega-9 is a key fatty acid when it comes to mineral absorption. Sufficient levels of oleic acid enhance absorption of minerals and fat soluble vitamins. Without high enough levels of it, you cannot absorb minerals like calcium and zinc. The following foods contain these types of fatty acids:

- → **Omega-3s:** wild-caught seafood (i.e., sardines, salmon, cod, shrimp, crab, etc.), grass-fed beef
- → **Omega-9s:** olive oil, avocados, almonds, almond oil, high-oleic safflower oil

ZINC

Zinc is needed for the catalytic activity of approximately 100 enzymes. (Enzymes jumpstart specific biochemical reactions.) Because of this, zinc plays an important role in balancing hormones. Zinc deficiency is a common culprit of hormonal acne. Zinc inhibits an enzyme called *5-alpha reductase, the enzyme that converts testosterone into its* active form, dihydrotestosterone (DHT).

Consequently, when zinc levels are low, your skin can be more susceptible to acne because you have higher levels of DHT circulating in your blood. We will talk more about this in the chapter on hormonal imbalances.

It is important to note that zinc is a key player in immune function. Primarily, zinc develops and activates T cell lymphocytes (T cells), which are critical to immune function. As part of the immune system, T cells actively search out and find infected cells and then destroy them. They also signal other immune cells to participate in the immune system response and further increase cellular activity.

Zinc also has antioxidant effects, and zinc *deficiency interferes with* the conversion of ALA (an important omega-3 fatty acid) into EPA and DHA. Zinc is needed to properly maintain levels of vitamin E and also aids in the absorption of vitamin A. These two vitamins assist in the reduction of scarring and inflammation and also increase immune cells. Long story short, zinc is a major immune system player because of its role in balancing hormones, fighting infections, and reducing inflammation.

The Standard American Diet (or SAD) is high in grains, processed foods, and foods that are devoid of nutrients. These grains can block absorption of some of our nutrients. Specifically, phytates are chemicals found in grains that can block absorption of nutrients. In order to increase zinc in your diet, consider increasing your intake of the following foods:

→ Oysters
→ Red meat
→ Poultry
→ Beans
→ Cashews
→ Almonds

VITAMIN A

Vitamin A deficiency is common amongst acne sufferers. A common medication used for treating severe acne, Accutane (isotretinoin), is a synthetic form of vitamin A. Vitamin A works by regulating prostaglandins that control sebum production in the skin.

Vitamin A also boosts the immune system—in fact, it's your first line of defense against invading viral, bacterial, and parasitic infections because it supports the mucosal barriers that line the intestinal barrier, respiratory system, and oral cavity. Vitamin A is also involved in producing antibodies and activating white blood cells in the immune system.

You can incorporate the following foods into your diet in order to increase your levels of vitamin A. But a warning! It's really important to eat the active forms of vitamin A, which are retinol, retinal, retinoic acid, and retinyl palmitate. You can only get the active form of vitamin A from eating animal products.

Plant sources have beta carotene, which is not biologically active vitamin A. Your body has to go through several steps to convert beta carotene into the active form of vitamin A. (Beta carotene is what you find in carrots and other vegetables.)

Here are foods that are high in active vitamin A:

→ Egg yolks
→ Beef liver
→ Butter
→ Salmon
→ Cod liver oil
→ Chicken liver

VITAMIN B6

Vitamin B6 is another common deficiency in acne sufferers. It is involved in 112 known enzymatic functions that primarily focus on protein metabolism. This vitamin not only helps us utilize protein, it aids in both fat and carbohydrate metabolism. A deficiency in vitamin B6 causes more uptake of and sensitivity to testosterone and impairs conversion of ALA to EPA and DHA.

Women who notice breakouts in correlation with their menstrual cycle are often deficient in this nutrient.

Vitamin B6 is also an essential cofactor in neurotransmitter synthesis. These are chemicals in the brain that regulate our mood. Some neurotransmitters that require vitamin B6 in order to be produced are serotonin, dopamine, histamine, GABA, and glycine.

A clinical trial published in *Nutrition Journal* in 2014 reported that high doses of B vitamins have been successful in improving mood states in both clinical and non-clinical populations.[1] Since acne sufferers tend to have higher levels of stress, B vitamins are very important for them to achieve good health. Always check with your practitioner for the appropriate dose to take. On your own, however, you can start with foods that are high in B6 and other B vitamins. Some good food sources are:

- ➤ Banana
- ➤ Avocado
- ➤ Sweet potato with the skin
- ➤ Potatoes with the skin

1   Stough et al., Reducing Occupational Stress

→ Organ meats
→ Salmon
→ Chicken breast
→ Turkey breast
→ Sunflower seeds

VITAMIN D

Vitamin D is a major hormone that is responsible for a variety of critical functions in your body. No wonder vitamin D gets a lot of attention in the medical field! Not only is it essential for bone health, this vitamin has been shown to have profound effects on balancing the immune system and regulating a type of white blood cell called T regulatory cells. For this reason, vitamin D is especially helpful when treating a lot of autoimmune conditions.

Vitamin D is also involved in maintaining a healthy intestinal barrier. This is significant, because a compromised intestinal barrier can be a gateway to inflammation. Vitamin D is a really important nutrient for maintaining that barrier between your bloodstream and the outside world. Maintaining the intestinal barrier also helps prevent a condition called leaky gut. (If you are not familiar with leaky gut, don't worry—we'll cover this topic more in the next chapter.) In addition to maintaining gut health, vitamin D has been shown to increase production of antimicrobial proteins that kill acne-causing bacteria in skin pores.[2]

It is worth noting that acne often becomes worse during the winter months due to vitamin D deficiency—it's exacer-

2 Nakatsuji et al., Sebum Free Fatty Acids Enhance The Innate Immune Defense

bated during times of the year when there isn't much sunlight. Even in the summer, our sedentary lifestyles and lack of outdoor activity make decreased levels vitamin D more likely. This vitamin is primarily obtained through sunlight (and is also found in some foods), so the best way to make sure you have sufficient levels of vitamin D is to schedule having regular outdoor time! Get 20 minutes of sun exposure per day without sunscreen. If you live in a climate or geographical location where regular sunlight exposure is not possible, you can purchase a sun lamp and use it for 20 minutes daily.

Although many doctors have warned people to stay out of the sun, adequate exposure is a necessity. The risks from sun exposure come into play when you stay out too long and get burned. You should never stay in the sunlight long enough to burn! It's also worth knowing that a diet that is high in antioxidants helps protect skin from the negative effects of sun exposure.

Believe it or not, some people are not able to get healthy levels of vitamin D into their cells from foods *or supplementation*—sun exposure is the only way they can get it.

Food sources of vitamin D mainly come from animal sources, including:

- → Sockeye salmon
- → Trout
- → Cod liver oil
- → Dried mushrooms

VITAMIN E

Vitamin E is known for its antioxidant and anti-inflammatory effects. Antioxidants protect cells from the damaging effects of free radicals by inhibiting lipid peroxidation. That's important, because free radicals damage cells and can increase the likelihood of inflammation. Also, because vitamin E is most abundant in sebum, vitamin E prevents lipid peroxidation in skin pores and the subsequent inflammation that leads to acne breakouts. Vitamin E works synergistically with vitamin A.

The following foods can be very effective at increasing your vitamin E levels:

+ Sunflower oil, sunflower seeds
+ Almonds
+ Hazelnuts
+ Avocados
+ Dark leafy greens
+ Butternut squash
+ Kiwi fruit

SELENIUM

Selenium is a trace element and a potent antioxidant, and it is also another mineral that is deficient in many acne sufferers. Its main role is to help recycle other antioxidants, specifically glutathione, alpha lipoic acid, vitamin C, and vitamin E. Selenium is also involved in thyroid function—the enzyme that converts the thyroid hormone into its active form needs selenium. Low thyroid function can be an acne trigger in some people, but we'll talk about that more in a later chapter.

Dietary sources of selenium include:

➜ Brazil nuts, mixed nuts
➜ Whole eggs, cooked
➜ Oysters
➜ Fish
➜ Organ meats
➜ Red meat
➜ Poultry

CHROMIUM

Chromium is most important for its potent effects on regulating blood sugar, namely that it helps prevent insulin resistance, which is common in people who have acne. In many acne sufferers, blood sugar balance impaired, leading to hormone imbalance, excess sebum production, and inflammation. That's why acne is often referred to as "diabetes of the skin."

Chromium content in foods varies. Due to varied farming and manufacturing processes, it's difficult to get chromium reliably from food sources. Some research studies have shown broccoli to be a good source.

NIACINAMIDE

Niacinamide (also known as vitamin B3) has many positive benefits for acne patients. It is anti-inflammatory, improves the skin barrier, shrinks the follicles, and reduces the risk of skin cancer by decreasing inflammation. It is a crucial nutrient, interacting with 400 enzymes in order to catalyze various reactions in the body. It synthesizes fatty acids and cholesterol and is critical in maintaining cellular antioxidant function.

Some rich food sources of niacin are:

➔ Mushrooms
➔ Potatoes
➔ Organ meats

BIOTIN

Biotin helps regulate sebum production and is known for its ability to promote the growth of skin cells. It also plays an important role in fat and carbohydrate metabolism.

Some foods that contain biotin are:

➔ Beef liver
➔ Legumes
➔ Whole eggs, cooked
➔ Fish
➔ Pork

You might be thinking that it might be difficult to incorporate these foods into your diet, but I promise you, it isn't! I have developed a couple of recipes specifically to help my patients get started. They are easy to make, you can take them on the road, and they contain a high volume of the nutrients I recommend.

The more you learn, the more you will understand that healing your skin can be fun! And delicious, too—the foods that are best for you also taste great.

> **Bonus Feature: For supplements suggestions**
> **to start getting these nutrients in,**
> **check out my radiant skin bundle at:**
> www.wellaheadchicago.com/blog/radiant

FACTORS THAT PREDISPOSE PEOPLE TO HAVING VITAMIN AND/ OR MINERAL DEFICIENCIES

Below are some lifestyle choices and stages in life that can predispose us to nutritional deficiencies by lowering our intake of nutrients, increasing our demand for them, compromising our ability to absorb them, accelerating our depletion of them, etc.

- Alcohol consumption
- Aging
- Impaired digestive health/poor nutrient absorption
- Medication (many medications cause nutrient depletion)
- Physical activity/weight training
- Pregnancy
- Smoking
- Food choices, special diets
- Stress

FOOD CHOICES THAT CAN IMPAIR NUTRITIONAL STATUS

Let's think of a common scenario that happens to all of us: your co-worker calls in sick, and your boss asks you to work overtime. You comply while fantasizing in the back of your mind about the food that you will pick up on the way home. Mmm...a burger and fries! That sounds so good. Even though the network crashes, you still manage to finish the project on time. Your stress levels, however, go through the roof! On the way home, not only do you get the burger and fries, but you add a shake. Why? Well, because you deserve it, right?

Let's take a look at how—when committing to heal acne in particular—we can give ourselves what we truly need to optimize our health rather than rewarding ourselves with what we crave. The following factors impair nutritional status and are well worth avoiding:

1. REACHING FOR STRESS FOODS

You want to make sure that you choose foods carefully during times of stress. We can all agree that one of the hardest parts about staying healthy is the timing and balance of our meals and snacks. All of us want to lead a normal life, but unfortunately, reaching for fast food defeats the healing process. The nutrition staff from the Center for Science in the Public Interest (CSPI)[3] warns us about some of the worst foods we can consume from grocery stores and restaurant chains. Some examples given were:

- ➜ Frozen pot pies
- ➜ Canned soups
- ➜ Most ready-made pizzas
- ➜ Lasagnas
- ➜ Blended coffee drinks
- ➜ Gourmet ice creams
- ➜ Fast-food milk shakes

3 10 Worst Foods | Center for Science in the Public Interest, 2020

2. UNCONTROLLED SUGAR CRAVINGS

High-glycemic foods promote inflammation and lead to diabetes, tooth decay, heart disease, and obesity. Drinks and sodas with added sugars—including fruit juices!—are still the number-one culprit of sugar consumption in the US.

So how can we control our sugar cravings? Planning ahead is important in order to make healthy choices on a consistent basis.

➜ Take time each week (preferably on the same day of the week) to plan your meals and snacks. Create your shopping list ahead of time and base it on healthy choices. Think about the places you will go and the foods you may need to carry with you all week long.
➜ Pack your lunch instead of eating out.
➜ Prep your vegetables in advance and store them in your refrigerator.

Planning a healthy breakfast that is not based on sugary treats will help stabilize your blood sugar throughout the day. You might also want to carry your own water bottle, because otherwise, when you find yourself thirsty and are on the go, you might wind up drinking something with sugar that you will regret later on.

3. THE STANDARD AMERICAN DIET

When it comes to choosing foods that aid in the acne-healing process, the Standard American Diet does not work in our favor. Many of us are eating a lot of refined carbohydrates, processed grains, foods that are high in sugar, fried foods,

foods high in fat, and other processed foods. (And not nearly enough fruits and vegetables.) Not only are these foods low in vitamins and minerals, grains contain chemicals called phytates that can actually block mineral absorption. If you're mostly eating grains, then you're creating nutritional deficiencies for yourself. In order to heal acne, you really have to do a diet overhaul and make a daily commitment to consuming a variety of vegetables, fruits, and other nutrient-dense foods.

4. SPECIAL DIETS

In my practice, I have seen that following any sort of special diet and thus eliminating an entire food group can predispose you to certain nutritional deficiencies. Let's talk about vegan diets as an example. Vitamin B12 is a deficiency most vegans are aware of. Most people who avoid meat or follow a vegan diet know to supplement with B12. (If you're deficient in vitamin B12, you can develop a condition called pernicious anemia where your body is not able to properly oxygenate your tissues.) However, there are some other vitamin deficiencies that are common in people following a vegan diet.

One of those is choline, another important nutrient and found primarily in eggs and liver. Choline is involved with metabolizing fat and supporting liver function—it actually protects your liver from developing fatty liver disease. The mineral zinc is found primarily in oysters, red meat, and poultry. Zinc has a lot of different functions, including being an antioxidant and supporting the immune system. Vitamin D is anti-inflammatory, supports your immune system, and plays a very big role in regulating blood sugar. It's also mostly only found in animal foods. Often, a lack of vitamin D can be one of the reasons why people who are vegan have issues with blood sugar regulation.

PUTTING THE INGREDIENTS TOGETHER

As you can see, several of the valuable nutrients described above are *exactly the nutrients we have talked about that you need* to eat in order to heal acne. I urge you to be conscious about choosing a special diet and to first seek the advice of a holistic doctor. If you do choose to limit your diet (or suspect that you have vitamin deficiencies for any other reason), I recommend having tests done to determine your vitamin and mineral levels. We will further discuss testing in a later chapter.

ARE YOU READY TO GET STARTED?

Now that you have read about which foods are "acne-friendly," you can get started with your own meal planning and design your own list of foods to shop for.

Proper functioning of the digestive system is imperative! If you have acne, you need to focus on foods that are nutrient-dense and that lower inflammation and promote healthy digestion. Poor digestion can cause nutritional deficiencies; conversely, digestive function can also be affected by nutritional deficiencies.

We assimilate nutrients through the villi, or the fingerlike projections in the small intestine. These increase the surface of the small intestine and enhance absorbtion of nutrients. When body chemistry is abnormal, the food that we ingest stagnates and ferments in the small intestine. This can often result in symptoms like bloating, gas, constipation or diarrhea, or even worse, Irritable Bowel Syndrome (IBS). Leaky gut can also be caused by nutritional deficiencies and can in turn cause malabsorption.

We must be able to absorb all of the nutrients we've discussed. Certain nutrients can even help repair the lining of the intestine. This is very important! The small intestine is literally a twenty-three-foot-long carpet. Imagine if you could walk on that carpet and make sure it was in good shape...! While you may not be able to actually do that, with the right program, those twenty-three feet can work *for you* instead of against you. In the next chapter, we will build this critical aspect of healing acne into your program.

Amanda's Story

Amanda had been dealing with acne since her late twenties. She tried making some changes to her diet and limited junk food and incorporated more vegetables. While making those changes did help, she was still noticing some breakouts. Amanda was lucky in the sense that she did not have severe acne—hers was very mild. Still, it was enough to be a nuisance. On top of acne, Amanda was dealing with brain fog and a lot of digestive discomfort. Deep down, she knew something was off with her entire body, and she wanted to have an individualized plan for healing.

Upon assessing Amanda's nutritional status, she did not have any clinical nutritional deficiencies, but she did have borderline deficiencies in a few key nutrients, and those had everything to do with her acne breakouts: chromium, magnesium, vitamin B3 (niacin). We have already talked about healthy levels of chromium and zinc are essential for blood sugar balance and how zinc is needed for hormone balance. Magnesium is a key player in balancing blood sugar also. If we had done conventional lab tests that only checked for a few vitamins and minerals in her serum (for example, B12, vitamin D, and iron), we would never have gotten this incredibly valuable insight that helped tailor her wellness blueprint. After three months of following her regimen, not only had Amanda's skin significantly improved, but she couldn't remember the last time she had had digestive discomfort. She was also feeling a lot less stressed.

CHAPTER FOUR

THE ROLE OF DIGESTIVE HEALTH IN ACNE

"You are not nourished by the food you eat, but in proportion to the amount you digest and assimilate."

~HERBERT SHELTON

I invite you to take this self-assessment quiz on digestive health. Please answer either "yes" or "no" to the following:

- ➤ Does your abdomen bloat after eating?
- ➤ Do you experience food allergies?
- ➤ Do you have consistent constipation and/or diarrhea?
- ➤ Do you have gas immediately following eating?
- ➤ Do you feel fullness one to three hours after eating?
- ➤ Do you have abdominal cramps?
- ➤ Do you have chronic urinary tract infections?
- ➤ Do you have foul-smelling stool?

→ Is there blood or mucus in your stools?

→ Do you have a history of antibiotic use?

As an acne sufferer, if you answered "yes" to even one of these questions, this chapter will be insightful for you. If you answered "yes" to more than a third of the questions, working to optimize your digestive health may be the solution to many of the problems you struggle with.

"Gut health" has become a buzz phrase lately for good reason—healthy digestion and a healthy gut are in fact central to optimal health. Problems in the digestive tract have far-reaching effects throughout the body and can be involved in a wide array of health concerns, such as diabetes, thyroid disorders, heart disease, mood disorders, neurological disorders, obesity, gynecologic disorders, skin disorders, etc.

Our skin is the largest organ in our body. It is inextricably linked with our digestive tract because they share a common embryologic origin. This correlation is often referred to as the "gut-skin axis." A chronic skin condition like acne is caused by multiple factors, and digestive health is a major contributing factor that simply cannot be ignored.

BEYOND DIGESTIVE SYMPTOMS

While symptoms like diarrhea, constipation, and indigestion can be indicators of gut health, even when there's a problem, those symptoms aren't always present. Symptoms are not always the best indicators of health—in fact, imbalances in digestive health are often present without any digestive symptoms. Another thing to keep in mind is that in our society, we have become accustomed to mediocre digestive function. We may not even realize that what we're experiencing on a day-to-day basis is not optimal. The digestive system directly and indirectly impacts many aspects of how the body functions, and all of that can impact skin health.

HOW GUT HEALTH AFFECTS ACNE

This is a loaded question that I'm sure you probably have if you are reading this book. I will do my best to answer it. To start, medical research has firmly established that there is a relationship between the health of the gut microbiome and acne. For those who are not familiar with the term, the "gut microbiome" is the population of microbes that are found in our digestive tract. These microbes must be kept in proper balance in order to maintain health. When they are not kept in proper balance, dysbiosis results.

Dysbiosis is an imbalance in the microbiome of the digestive tract that is significant enough to negatively impact health. It typically involves an increase in bad microbes and a decrease in good microbes, but it's not always that black-and-white—there are definitely grey areas. Good microbes and normal flora can also do damage when they are not kept in the appropriate proportions. Dysbiosis can have varying levels of severity. For many acne sufferers, courses of antibiotics are a precipitating factor. When certain organisms overgrow, they can also cause food allergies.

KEY FACTORS THAT CORRELATE ACNE AND GUT HEALTH

When digestion is not optimal, it has a domino effect on each of the subsequent factors:

→ **Nutrient absorption:** Nutritional status is the foundation of good health. When digestion is less than optimal and the intestinal barrier is damaged, this can interfere with our ability to assimilate macronutrients (carbs, protein, fat) and micronutrients (vitamins, minerals, etc.).

→ **Hormone balance:** Sluggish digestion and elimination can interfere with liver function and hormone balance. Imbalances in the gut microbiome can interfere with blood sugar control.

→ **Leaky gut:** When the barrier between your digestive tract and your bloodstream is not intact, it gives way to systemic inflammation. Larger molecules are able to cross the intestinal barrier and toxins produced by bacteria can enter the bloodstream.

→ **Food sensitivities:** Low digestive function can lead to food sensitivities if proteins that are normally broken down can instead enter the bloodstream and trigger an immune response. Protein maldigestion causes food allergies. We'll talk about this more in a later chapter.

> "The lines of communication, as mediated by gut microbes, may be direct and indirect—ultimately influencing the degree of acne by a systemic effect on inflammation, oxidative stress, glycemic control, tissue lipid levels, pathogenic

bacteria, as well as levels of neuropeptides and mood-regulating neurotransmitters. There appears to be more than enough supportive evidence to suggest that gut microbes, and the integrity of the gastrointestinal tract itself, are contributing factors in the acne process." Excerpt from Gut Pathogens, 2011

WHAT CAUSES DYSBIOSIS

When acne is present, there is a chronic low-grade infection. Some common causes of dysbiosis are:

→ **Diet choices:** Foods high in sugar and simple carbohydrates can feed the growth of bad bacteria and fungus in the microbiome

→ **Digestive dysfunction:** Digestion is a complex and intricate process, and when there is a breakdown in any of the steps during digestion, this can set the stage for dysbiosis

→ **Toxins**

→ **Medications**, especially antibiotics and medications that decrease stomach acid production

→ **Pathogens**: Bad microbes that cause serious illness

→ **Stress:** High cortisol levels can shift the composition of the gut microbiome

→ **Sleep deprivation**

HOW DYSBIOSIS DAMAGES HEALTH

Dysbiosis has far-reaching effects throughout the body that go beyond the gut:

➔ Dysbiosis damages the intestinal lining

➔ Dysbiosis promotes inflammation and autoimmune issues

➔ Dysbiosis produces harmful byproducts, namely an overgrowth of bad microbes that can cause an accumulation of toxic byproducts that can then circulate in the bloodstream, causing inflammation

➔ Dysbiosis can cause low digestive function, which can create the perfect environment for dysbiosis and bacterial overgrowth and therefore lead to food sensitivities

➔ Dysbiosis decreases levels of beneficial microbes

ALCOHOL IS NOT YOUR FRIEND

There are different categories of toxins, alcohol being one of them. Alcohol promotes overgrowth of yeast as well as bacteria that produce a toxin called lipopolysaccharide (LPS). We'll talk about LPS more later in this chapter. Alcohol has also been shown to disrupt the tight junctions between the epithelial cells that form the intestinal barrier, which causes leaky gut. Think of alcohol as a double-whammy.

DIGESTION IS A COORDINATED CHAIN OF EVENTS

If there is a breakdown in any of the following steps, it can cause problems:

➔ Mastication (chewing)

➔ Swallowing

- Secretion of digestive enzymes
- Digestion
- Absorption
- Peristalsis (contractions in the gut that stimulate bowel movements)

LOW STOMACH ACID

Up to 40% of acne sufferers have low stomach acid (called hypochlorhydria).[4] This sets the stage for bacteria overgrowth in the small intestine (SIBO) because bacteria are then able to travel from the colon into the small intestine, where levels of bacteria are meant to be exponentially lower compared to the colon.

> *"Although the frequency of SIBO in acne vulgaris has not yet been investigated, a recent report indicates that SIBO is ten times more prevalent in those with acne rosacea vs. healthy controls. Correction of SIBO leads to marked clinical improvement in patients with rosacea."*[5]

Stomach acid is our first line of defense against foreign invaders. Low stomach acid can create the perfect landscape for infections to take hold and acne to develop. This certainly be a major contributing factor to acne. Keep in mind that the root cause of hypochlorhydria is caused by a deeper problem. Common causes of hypochlorhydria include hypothyroidism, antacid medications, proton pump inhibitor medications, chronic stress, and chronic low-grade infections. When stom-

4   Bowe and Logan, "Acne vulgaris, probiotics and the gut-brain-skin axis"
5   Smith et al., "A Low Glycemic Load Diet Improves Symptoms in Acne Vulgaris Patients"

ach acid production is low, the entire chain of events during digestion is impacted: digestive enzyme production and the movement of bowels are affected, and you may wind up with indigestion as well. The benefits of having proper levels of stomach acid are why some people notice improvement in acne when they start taking apple cider vinegar.

Poor digestive function can be caused by several factors: medications, certain medical conditions, and chronic low-grade infections can all affect the activity of the vagus nerve. This nerve is responsible for stimulating the chain of events that are necessary for digestive function, from stimulating the release of digestive enzymes to causing bowel movements. Being in a state of chronic stress can decrease activity of the vagus nerve by causing an imbalance between your sympathetic and parasympathetic nervous systems, causing your body to be in a perpetual state of fight-or-flight. (Our parasympathetic nervous system is responsible for our rest-and-digest mode, while our sympathetic nervous system triggers fight-or-flight.)

Propionibacterium acnes is the bacteria that gets all the focus in terms of causing acne, but several other microbes can cause acne and have been cultured from acne lesions: streptococcus, pseudomonas, klebsiella, proteus, pityrosporum, and yeast. Tetracycline causes proliferation of these microbes, and overgrowth of these bacteria is common after antibiotic use. In addition, it's not only bacteria that can cause acne—yeast overgrowth and parasites can also cause acne by disrupting the gut microbiome.

If you suffer from recurrent yeast infections, it's reasonable to suspect that yeast may also be playing a role in your acne. Candida is a normal flora that is found in the digestive tract in a healthy person. The problem comes when there's overgrowth. Nowadays, there's more awareness around Candida albicans overgrowth, but other species of candida can cause acne, as can other types of fungi.

PARASITES

Parasites are a less-often-acknowledged cause of acne. Some people may think parasites are only a concern if you're traveling to a developing country, but parasites are relatively common in the United States. In fact, it's estimated that millions of Americans are affected by parasites, in part because poor digestive function creates an ideal environment for parasites to take hold. One may be exposed to a parasite from time to time through water, undercooked meat, pets, etc. *If your digestive function is healthy,* you produce enough stomach acid, you have a normal frequency of bowel movements, and you have a healthy intestinal lining, this serves as a layer of protection against parasites.

NORMAL FLORA

Good bacteria produce a protective coating that is needed to protect the intestinal barrier. Certain strains of beneficial bacteria also produce a short-chain fatty acid called butyrate. Butyrate is the preferred fuel of the cells that form the intestinal barrier; these cells also need butyrate to regenerate themselves. Not having enough good bacteria in your digestive tract can be just as problematic as having too much bad bacteria. This is because good bacteria perform some essential functions, like making B vitamins and vitamin K and producing butyrate and other necessary chemicals for healthy digestive function. When levels of good bacteria are too low, it gives bad bacteria room to grow and cause problems. When bad bacteria overgrow, they can release a chemical called lipopolysaccharide (LPS) into our bloodstream. LPS is found in the cell wall of some bacteria, and when it ends up in our bloodstream it can be highly inflammatory. This is referred to as metabolic endotoxemia, and it is a driving force behind metabolic disease.

CONSTIPATION/GUT MOTILITY

Acne sufferers have a higher risk of gastrointestinal problems. A study of 13,000 adolescents showed that those with acne were more likely to suffer from digestive health symptoms such as constipation, bad breath, acid reflux, and bloating.[6] Poor digestive function can cause chronic constipation, which can be a major obstacle to good health—if you're constipated, your body cannot properly detoxify itself.

PROBIOTICS, ANYONE?

"Can I take a probiotic or drink bone broth to heal my gut?" This is a question I've heard many times. Hopefully after reading this chapter, you'll have a better understanding of why the answer is not that simple.

In order to effectively correct a problem, you have to first identify it. While a number of supplements and natural rem-

6   Zhang et al., "Risk factors for sebaceous gland diseases and their relationship to gastrointestinal dysfunction in adolescents"

edies have been popularized as being beneficial for digestive health, general recommendations for digestive health may or may not benefit you as an individual. As an example, products like collagen and bone broth are generally recommended for healing leaky gut, but they may or may not benefit you if you don't know the underlying cause of YOUR leaky gut. Collagen and bone broth could even make your symptoms worse if you are *not deficient in glutamine and are taking it in a* concentrated form. Similarly, a probiotic formula may or may not be helpful if you don't know anything about the balance of bacteria in your digestive tract.

TESTS THAT ARE HELPFUL IN ASSESSING GUT HEALTH

There are a number of tests available, so it's important to discuss with your health care provider which test(s) will be most valuable based on your health concerns. Because there are several aspects to optimizing gut health, a personalized approach is needed. Identifying specific factors that are affecting your digestive health will help you enhance your digestive health with certainty and within a shorter period of time. Here are a few tests I've found to be useful:

- ➤ Intestinal permeability
- ➤ Food allergies
- ➤ Stool testing
- ➤ Vitamin/mineral analysis
- ➤ SIBO breath testing
- ➤ Organic acids

Erica's Story

Erica had been struggling with severe cystic acne ever since she had finished college and entered the workforce. Her first job was as a nurse working the night shift, and she had very different hours than what her body was used to! Shortly after beginning her position, she started to struggle with severe cystic acne.

Over the course of the next few years, she felt like she had tried everything she could to get rid of it—she had gone through most of what conventional medicine had to offer and had tried many different skin care products. By the time she came to see me, she felt like she was running out of options. The only thing left for her to try was Accutane, but because of its known side effects, she wasn't keen on that idea.

After talking to Erica and getting a deeper understanding of her struggle and where she was in her journey, we decided we really needed to dig deeper to find out what was going on with her body and where her imbalances were. Evaluating her gut health would be a key part of that.

When we got the results of her stool test results back, it was apparent that she was dealing with a severe imbalance in her microbiome that more than likely would have been missed with conventional lab tests. Her normal bacterial flora were out of balance—she had too few of some species and too many of others. She had high levels of some problematic bacteria and various species of candida (yeast), and a parasite was also present. Based on what lab results revealed, it was evident that the probiotics she had been taking were not helping, because they were the wrong formula for her individual microbiome imbalance. Fortunately, she could correct some of her key problems with the right supplements and lifestyle changes.

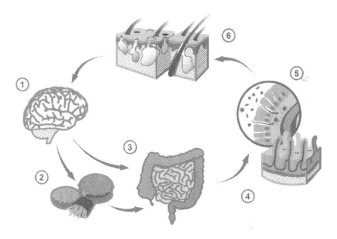

FIGURE 1—POTENTIAL PATHWAYS OF THE GUT-BRAIN-SKIN AXIS IN ACNE VULGARIS:

Psychological stress by itself or combined with junk foods shifts the composition of the gut microbiome in a negative direction. This can lead to a leaky gut as the protective coating produced by good bacteria is lost and toxins produced by bad microbes can leak into the bloodstream causing inflammation. This chain of events causes excess sebum production and acne flares.

CHAPTER FIVE

LIVER FUNCTION AND DETOXIFICATION

"The person who takes medicine must recover twice, once from the disease and once from the medicine."

~WILLIAM OSLER

I invite you to take this self-assessment quiz . Please answer either "yes" or "no" to the following:

- ➜ Do you have an intolerance to greasy foods?
- ➜ Do you have light or clay-colored stools?
- ➜ Is the odor of your sweat offensive?
- ➜ Do you have high cholesterol?
- ➜ Have you noticed a yellowish tint to the whites of your eyes?
- ➜ How many times per week do you drink alcohol?
- ➜ Are you easily intoxicated if you drink wine?

➤ Do you have sensitivity to chemicals (perfumes, cleaning agents, etc.)?

➤ Have you used any prescription medications long-term?

As an acne sufferer, if you answered "yes" to even one of these questions, this chapter will be insightful for you. If you answered "yes" to more than a third of the questions, detoxification and supporting liver function may be a solution to many of the problems you struggle with.

When we think of detoxification, most of us think of the liver, and rightfully so. However, the skin is another major organ of detoxification, particularly if our liver is struggling to function properly—when our toxic burden gets to a level beyond what our body can tolerate, toxins can come out in our skin because this is one of the ways the body discharges and excretes them. Toxins burden our detoxification systems, shift our microbiome out of balance, cause leaky gut, and disrupt our hormone balance. You probably won't be surprised to learn that impaired liver function is very common among acne sufferers.

MAIN FUNCTIONS OF THE LIVER

Healthy liver function is essential for general health and well-being. The liver has over 500 known metabolic functions. It plays a role in digestion, regulating blood sugar, the endocrine system, and protein and fat metabolism. The liver is also responsible for making a substance called bile. Bile is stored in the gallbladder and is essential for proper digestion and absorption of fat as well as fat-soluble vitamins.

The liver is one of our major body organs that manages our exposure to toxins and processes and eliminates toxic waste from the body. It does this by converting many of these toxins into a form that can be easily excreted through our urine or our stool. Unfortunately, the amount of toxic chemicals that we are all exposed to in our day-to-day living poses certain health risks. In fact, many people have been pushed beyond the limit of what their body can tolerate.

What the liver does:

→ Assists digestion
→ Metabolizes drugs, vitamins, and hormones
→ Stores vitamins and minerals
→ Stores toxins
→ Stores glycogen and triglycerides
→ Filters our blood
→ Converts vitamin D into its active form
→ Metabolizes fat and makes cholesterol, lipoproteins, and phospholipids
→ Produces bile (which is needed for digestion and absorption of fat)
→ Performs Phase I & Phase 2 detoxification
→ Balances hormones
→ Gets rid of toxins
→ Neutralizes toxins
→ Produces carnitine
→ Produces amino acids (the building blocks of proteins)

TOXINS

The amount of chemicals we are exposed to in our environment is at an all-time high.

A study done by the Environmental Working Group in 2005 revealed an average of 200 industrial chemicals and pollutants in the umbilical cord blood of newborn infants: pesticides, consumer product ingredients, gasoline, wastes from coal burning, etc. These shocking statistics underscore the fact that most of us are beginning our lives with a significant toxic burden. This places a tremendous amount of stress on the liver and our detoxification system. Some toxins we commonly come across are:

→ Drugs (prescription, OTC, recreational, alcohol)Food additives
→ Cosmetic additives
→ Agricultural chemicals
→ Pollutants
→ Household chemicals

When the toxic burden is too high, it can precipitate various symptoms and problems like skin problems, digestive problems, allergies, headaches, fatigue, and joint pain. In many ways, we have been conditioned to think that most health problems are caused by genetics and that our genetics determine our health. However, there has been an exponential increase in allergies and autoimmune issues over the past five decades. A purely genetic cause would not account for this drastic increase. There is mounting evidence that this increase is due to industrialization and the increasing amounts of chemicals we are being exposed to on a daily basis.

IT'S NOT JUST ACNE

HOW LIVER FUNCTION IS RELATED TO ACNE

The million-dollar question is "How does impaired liver function relate to acne?" If we take a look at the functions of the liver, we can easily see the connections. Let's take metabolism of fat as an example. A high-fat diet can lead to impaired fat metabolism, which can result in oily skin that is more prone to breakouts. Do you see the domino effect? It goes back to the concept of nutrient deficiencies we talked about in Chapter Three. Pantothenate (also known as vitamin B5) and carnitine are involved in fat metabolism in the liver. When fat metabolism is optimal and these nutrients are at healthy levels in the body, they are able to properly assist with the conversion of fats we consume by converting them into energy sources. Consequently, there is then less sebum production in the skin and a reduced pore size...and a reduced risk of acne breakouts.

When we consume a high-fat diet, our need for vitamin B5 and carnitine increases, so we become more likely to develop a deficiency of them. When this happens, there is more sebum production in the skin and the sebum has a thicker texture that clogs pores...which then more readily leads to acne. The amount and quality of fat in your diet has an impact on the chemical composition of your sebum.

ENDOCRINE DISRUPTORS AND
HORMONE IMBALANCE

Earlier, we touched on how the liver is involved in neutralizing toxins in Phase I and Phase II detoxification. We've also established that we are exposed to a wide variety of chemicals in the environment. When these enter our bodies, they can have profound negative effects on our health: they can promote inflammation by being a significant burden on our immune system, for example, and they can begin to act as hormones and interfere with hormone signaling and/or increase or decrease production of certain hormones.

Many of these chemicals can bind to the same receptor sites that our hormones bind to. For this reason, they are often referred to as xenohormones. Xenohormones (compounds produced outside the human body that mimic hormones) are endocrine disruptors because they can disrupt normal hormone balance. There are both synthetic and natural sources of xenohormones. For our purposes, we're going to focus on synthetic sources. We are exposed to these chemicals in our everyday lives, and we're probably not even aware of many of them—they're found in the air we breathe, in the food we eat, the water we drink, and sometimes even in our workplace (i.e., occupational exposures).

Some of the most prevalent endocrine disruptors are:

→ Bisphenol A
→ Dioxin
→ Atrazine
→ Perchlorate
→ Fire/flame retardants
→ Lead
→ Arsenic
→ Mercury
→ Perfluorinated chemicals
→ Organophosphate pesticides
→ Glycol ethers

If our exposure to these chemicals is too high and our liver function is not being properly supported in order to be able to manage and excrete these chemicals, this can have far-reaching effects throughout our body, whether that's an increased risk of cancer, reproductive problems, or obesity. Toxic load can also shift the gut microbiome, and disruption of hormone balance from chemicals can also exacerbate acne.

COMMON SOURCES OF EXPOSURE TO HORMONE-DISRUPTING CHEMICALS

These products are some of the sources of our biggest everyday exposure to chemicals. Here's where we can make adjustments to reduce our exposure:

- Personal care products
- Cosmetics
- Plastics
- Conventionally farmed meat
- Dry cleaning
- Air pollution
- Water pollution

It's important to reduce your exposure to toxins, especially from skin care and personal care products as they can be absorbed through the skin directly into the bloodstream.

HOW THE LIVER AND THE MICROBIOME ARE CONNECTED

The connection and communication between the gut and the liver is called the gut-liver axis. The gut-liver axis is affected by intestinal barrier health, intestinal dysbiosis, and migration of bacteria from the gut. Venous blood from the intestines drains into the portal vein in the liver, so the gut and the liver are connected through the circulatory system. Pathogens can travel from the gut to the liver through the portal vein and also through a compromised intestinal barrier. (Remember, alcohol disrupts tight junctions and makes us more prone to having leaky gut.) Gut dysbiosis puts additional stress on the liver, driving inflammation and compromising function.

In the previous chapter, we talked about the various microbes that can cause acne. The role that the liver plays with these microbes goes back to its role as a major organ of detoxification. Bacteria are absorbed from the colon into the liver, where specialized cells in the liver (called Kupffer cells) digest these bacteria in order to prevent them from entering the bloodstream.

Enter antibiotics and antifungals, which are commonly used to treat chronic urinary tract infections and bacterial vaginosis. However, the more they are used, the more they can cause problems in the long run. Antibiotics feed bacteria and yeast overgrowth and also put stress on the liver. Repetitive use causes antibiotics to build up in the liver, and this gives streptococcus the opportunity to build up resistance to antibiotics. (Streptococcus lives in the liver when there is an abundance of food there for them.) Streptococcus can adapt to the presence of antibiotics and start to use them as fuel.

Strep infections treated with antibiotics (strep throat, sties, sinus infections, etc.) lay the foundation for acne to develop later in life—as we touched on in Chapter Four, group A Strep (streptococcus pyogenes) is one of the types of bacteria that drives acne breakouts. Many acne sufferers have a history of taking antibiotics for non-acne conditions before they ever took any antibiotics for acne. And don't forget, we can also be exposed to antibiotics through our food supply.

> *"We have recently demonstrated that antibiotic therapy for acne when given topical and/or orally to young adults may profoundly affect an individual's likelihood of being colonized with group A streptococcus (GAS)..."*[7]

Strep loves to travel through the lymphatic system, the other circulatory system that rids our body of toxins. The lymphatic system also contains white blood cells that fight infections. Strep tends to take the path of least resistance, so it takes the lymphatic system when the system has become weakened and doesn't have as many lymphocytes to fight infections. This is believed to be one of the reasons why people can get breakouts on different parts of the body, whether it's the jawline, forehead, chest, back, or upper arms. Byproducts from dairy and eggs can accumulate in the subcutaneous tissue and provide fuel for streptococcus.

7 Margolis, David. "Acne And Group A Strep"

Kevin's Story

Kevin was in his late twenties when he came in to see me. He had never really struggled with acne as a teenager, but ever since he had moved to Chicago and started a new high-stress job, breakouts had been popping up.

I did a thorough intake with him and noticed some key areas where he could make lifestyle changes to reduce the stress on his digestive and detoxification systems and likely notice improvement in his skin quickly. One of those things was reducing his alcohol consumption. He was a very outgoing, social person, and he worked in sales, so taking clients out for dinner and drinks to close deals was part of his job. You can imagine that when I told him he would have to cut back on alcohol if he really wanted to see his skin improve, he felt like it was the end of the world.

I told him that if he felt like eliminating alcohol all at once was too much, he could start small by setting a SMART goal (Specific, Measurable, Attainable, Realistic, Time-oriented). He decided his goal would be that he would not keep any kind of alcohol in his home. He would partake in alcohol only when he was with clients, and he would limit himself to one drink. He would also find gluten-free substitutes for bread, pasta, cereal, etc. After one month, he noticed dramatic improvements in his skin. You see, not only does alcohol put additional stress on the liver, it also disrupts the tight junctions that keep the intestinal barrier intact.

CHAPTER SIX

HORMONAL BALANCE

"Everything we do affects our hormones,
which in turn affects everything we do."

~ROB SULAVER

I invite you to take this self-assessment quiz on hormonal balance. Please answer either "yes" or "no" to the following:

➜ Are you frequently experiencing sleep deprivation?
➜ Have you ever had mood swings that created problems with your daily functions?
➜ Do you experience intense sugar cravings?
➜ Do you notice that you have digestive issues like bloating, gas, or indigestion?
➜ Have you had difficulty losing or gaining weight?
➜ Do you feel constant fatigue?
➜ Are your stress levels above what your body can handle?
➜ Have you ever taken oral contraceptives?

➜ Do you suffer from depression or anxiety?

➜ Have you noticed hair loss?

➜ Do you have food allergies?

As an acne sufferer, if you answered "yes" to even one of these questions, this chapter will be insightful for you. If you answered "yes" to more than a third of the questions, working to balance your hormones may be the solution to many of the problems you struggle with.

The real question is "How do hormones cause acne?" The answer to this question will be slightly different in females compared to males, yet there will be a lot of similarities. Hormonal balance is like a house of cards—it is delicate and requires just the right positioning of each one to support all of the others. If you pull just one of the cards away, the whole tower falls. Much like the various nutrients discussed in Chapter Three, our hormones should work together seamlessly. There's a delicate balance that has to be maintained in order for the hormone system to function properly and fuel bodily functions. Unbalanced hormonal shifts give bacteria an opportunity to overtake the immune system.

TRIGGERS THAT PUT STRESS ON THE HORMONE SYSTEM

The following three factors can also be a chain of events. For example, first you experience a stressful event; then you eat junk/comfort food (which often contains high levels of sugar), which upsets the microbiome; then immunity becomes compromised. Consequently, hormones are imbalanced, and the cascading effect is acne.

- Overloading our systems with stress
- Overloading our systems with sugar
- Systemic inflammation

THE ROLE OF STRESS

To understand the effects of stress on acne, we first need to understand the physiologic implications of chronic stress. Please note that this is not an exhaustive list! I mainly want to highlight factors that have a direct impact on acne:

- Decrease in mucosal immunity
- Shifts in the microbiome
- Increased need for vitamins/minerals (B vitamins, magnesium, vitamin C)
- Decreased digestive function
- Reduced thyroid function
- Shifts in sex hormone levels
- Altered glucose metabolism
- Poor detoxification
- Increased storage of fat, difficulty losing weight
- Decreased sleep quality

Research studies have shown that psychological stress slows the movement of waste through the digestive tract, fosters an overgrowth of bacteria, and compromises the integrity of the intestinal barrier.[8]

If the state of stress is prolonged, then the effects of the resulting health problems can become magnified and lead to even greater health problems.

8 Smith et al., A low-glycemic-load diet improves symptoms in acne vulgaris patients

THE "ON" AND "OFF" BUTTONS FOR STRESS

The brain initiates our stress response. You might lose your wallet, or maybe you hear some devastating news about a family member. Immediately, your amygdala (located in the brain stem) receives this information, interprets it, and processes it. Upon perceiving danger, it quickly alerts the hypothalamus. While this emotional processing is still going on, the hypothalamus acts as the central commander and sends a clear order to the nervous system, telling it that you have one of two options: fight or flight.

The hypothalamus also communicates to the autonomic nervous system by controlling involuntary body functions like breathing, blood pressure, heartbeat, digestion, and the dilation or constriction of key blood vessels and small airways in the lungs. This system contains two components: the sympathetic nervous system and the parasympathetic nervous system. The sympathetic nervous system is the "on button" that responds to perceived dangers. The parasympathetic nervous system is the "off button" that calms the body down after the danger has passed.

If you've struggled with acne, I'm sure you've noticed how every time you've got some big event coming, whether it's a hot date, a job interview, or a party...you get a zit! We have our stress response to thank for this. During times of stress, our immune system becomes depressed and less able to fight infections.

The hormonal system comes into play when the hypothalamus activates the adrenal glands. These little orange-colored glands rest on top of the kidneys and are usually half an inch tall and three inches wide. The adrenals help *manage stress but are also damaged by stress.*

This is a very important point to remember when we are connecting the dots between digestive function, immunity, hormone balance, and stress. Two of the most immediate reactions to stress are that the adrenals produce three stress response hormones: cortisol, norepinephrine, and epinephrine. These glands respond by pumping the hormone epinephrine (more commonly known as adrenaline) into the bloodstream.

CORTISOL

Cortisol is our major stress hormone. Cortisol levels increase early in the morning to meet the demands of the day, and then they gradually decrease throughout the day, reaching their lowest point late in the evening through a pattern known as the circadian rhythm. Cortisol regulates immunity and enhances glucose production. *It also plays a crucial role in helping the body adapt to stress.* It's also worth pointing out that the gut becomes more permeable during times of stress.

Medical research abounds with definitive evidence on the connection between skin disorders (including acne) and stress. A study conducted at the College of Medicine, King Saudi University (KSU) between January and June of 2015 revealed significant increases in skin imbalances amongst a sample of 1,435 undergraduate students with heightened stress levels.

The study evaluated three groups of students: the least-stressed, the moderately-stressed and the most-stressed students. Noticeable changes in skin conditions occurred during exam weeks and also throughout the fourth and fifth years of medical school. Female students and older students of both genders suffered from more oily, waxy patches on the skin or scalp. When compared to less-stressed students, these highly-stressed students also experienced more rashes.

Electronic surveys monitored these female medical students during exam weeks and again throughout the fourth and fifth years of medical school. These periods were the highest-stress periods. When compared to the least-stressed students, highly-stressed students suffered from a much greater percentage of warts and pimples. Their scalps became flaky and some of them lost hair. Itchy hands were also common.

This evidence is not surprising to me since in medical school, I myself experienced some of these same symptoms. This is what led me to question medical treatment strategies more deeply—I knew that there had to be more options for acne sufferers than what allopathic (i.e., conventional) medicine offered.

THE LONG-TERM EFFECTS THAT STRESS CAUSES IF WE DO NOT LEARN HOW TO USE THE "OFF BUTTON"

In 2015, medical researchers from the Ireland School of Medicine, Ireland Teagasc Food Research Centre and the Department of Anatomy and Neuroscience, University College Cork in Ireland determined that the role stress plays in the gut and immune function can begin as early as adolescence. This may in fact set the stage for skin problems to develop as a teen or through young adulthood.

Environmental factors that disturb gut bacteria may affect gut-brain communication, altering the trajectory of brain development and increasing susceptibility to mental and emotional stress. In this same study, when mice were treated with antibiotics after weaning and onwards, their gut bacteria became disrupted. Sadly, they suffered from increased anxiety and cognitive deficits.

WHAT ELSE HAPPENS WHEN THE STRESS RESPONSE IS CHRONIC AND PROLONGED

Various dysfunctions occur when stress disrupts anabolism, a constructive phase during which the body uses metabolic energy derived from nutrients to repair, rejuvenate, and rebuild organs, cells, and tissues. This phase is restorative and occurs during the night. However, stress disrupts this crucial phase when catabolism (the supply of energy that makes all actions possible, right down to the cellular level) *overrides our capacity to restore all of our systems.*

THYROID HORMONES

The thyroid is a small ductal gland that weighs less than an ounce. It is located in front of the neck, just below the Adam's apple and along the trachea. The thyroid is important because it *interconnects the entire endocrine system.* It essentially acts as your body's thermostat and drives metabolic processes in the body. This means that the thyroid is a key player in the house of cards. Not surprisingly, thyroid dysfunction and acne often go hand in hand.

It's estimated that 20 million Americans have some form of thyroid condition and that 60% do not know it because they have not been properly tested. Even if they *are tested, only their TSH level is* tested, and this is not an adequate marker. This is why comprehensive testing is a must.

IS HORMONAL ACNE PURELY HORMONAL?

This is an area where more research needs to be done to enable the medical community to have a better understanding of acne. Some scientists believe that hormonal shifts—whether they are due to the menstrual cycle, puberty, stress, etc.—present opportunities for bacteria to travel more easily. For example, during hormonal shifts, lymphocytes (a type of white blood cell) are at their weakest, and strep can escape from the liver into the lymphatic system. The lymphocytes are able to kill some of the strep, but many of the cells can escape into the subcutaneous tissue just beneath the skin. This is a basically a skin eruption waiting to occur once other conditions are met. (We'll cover those other conditions later in this chapter.)

HORMONE BALANCE AND CONNECTING THE DOTS

Let's talk about how hormonal disruption is related to acne. Pay close attention to the different functions of these hormones—when you realize how many functions they have that relate to digestion, immunity, and the control of stress, you will understand how just pulling one of them away from your house of cards can cause a collapse.

These hormone imbalances can result in acne:

→ Hypothyroidism
→ Polycystic Ovarian Syndrome (PCOS)
→ Pre-diabetes/diabetes

An important point to keep in mind here is that people often have imbalances in their hormones that do not fit a medical diagnosis but can still cause them to have symptoms. Many who suffer from acne have hormone imbalances that are not severe enough to fit a diagnosis, for example, but if those imbalances are left untreated, that can eventually progress to a full-blown medical condition.

ESTROGEN

Estrogen stimulates breasts and reproductive organs and protects their functions. Estrogen is also your hormonal brain booster. It acts on neurotransmitters and affects cognitive factors such as learning and attention span, memory, mood, sleep, and libido. It preserves bone mass and also the elasticity of skin tone. (It ensures the moisture content of the skin.) Not only does it dilate blood vessels, it keeps plaque from forming in them. Interestingly, estrogen will also decrease the perception of pain.

PROGESTERONE

Progesterone is a companion to estrogen. The ovaries mainly produce it, but trace amounts are found in the adrenal glands, peripheral nerves, and brain cells. Along with estrogen, progesterone ensures the development and function of the breasts and female reproductive tract. Yet it has one function that estrogen does not: it acts on certain brain receptors to improve your sleep by causing sedation.

With respect to the impact progesterone has on acne, it is important to note that *progesterone increases sensitivity to insulin and helps thyroid hormones function. Progesterone* also helps us use our fat effectively. Because of this and because it lowers triglycerides, it blocks arterial plaque formation, thus helping the cardiovascular system. Fluctuations in progesterone levels occur during the menstrual cycle, and that's when many women experience breakouts.

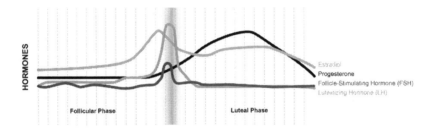

FIGURE 2

ANDROGENS

Androgens are a group of hormones that play a key role in reproductivity in males and females. The key androgens are testosterone, DHEA, and androstenedione. In females, androgens are also converted into estrogens. Androgens help regulate many organ functions outside of the reproductive tract, including the kidney, liver, bones, and muscles. Androgen excess can be a precursor of acne, and high levels of androgens can also be correlated with blood sugar problems.

TESTOSTERONE

Both men and women have testosterone, and it has a protective effect against cardiovascular disease in both men and women. (Women manufacture testosterone in the ovaries and adrenal glands.) Testosterone enhances libido and sexual response. It also strengthens ligaments, builds muscle and bone, assists with brain functioning, and is associated with assertive behavior and a sense of well-being. In both genders, testosterone levels influence both stamina and restful sleep. Again, fluctuating levels of this hormone are associated with acne in males, and high levels of androgens can be correlated to blood sugar problems.

DEHYDROEPIANDROSTERONE (DHEA)

DHEA is the most plentifully circulating hormone in our bodies. It is very important because it protects us against the effects of physical stress. It is produced in *both the ovaries and the adrenal glands*, and smaller quantities of DHEA are produced in the skin and the brain. Psychologically, it is indispensable—it increases a sense of well-being, decreases pain, and enhances immunity. It can be converted into its companion hormones, estrogen and progesterone.

THE GLYCEMIC INDEX AND ACNE

Acne is often referred to as "diabetes of the skin." In order to balance your hormones, you must balance your blood sugar. In conventional medicine, blood sugar is looked at in black-and-white terms—you either have diabetes/prediabetes or you don't—but in contrast, in holistic medicine, blood sugar is viewed through a different perspective. Rather than being a black-and-white issue, there is a grey area and a continuum of blood sugar control. By the time a person is diagnosed with diabetes, they have lost some function of their pancreas. People often have imbalances in their blood sugar that are much less severe than diabetes but *that can still cause acne and contribute to hormone imbalance.*

In a study done in July of 2007 on the glycemia/acne connection in young males, the American Journal of Clinical Nutrition reported a significant connection between a decrease in the glycemic index and a decrease in acne.

Forty-three male acne patients aged 15 through 25 participated in a 12-week assessment. After eating a low-glycemic-load diet of 25% energy from protein and 45% from low-glycemic-index carbohydrates, their acne lesion counts and their acne severity decreased by 23%. In addition, the young males in the study lost weight. This article concluded that following a low-glycemic-load diet as well as altering nutrition-related lifestyle factors reduced acne in the young male population.

When it comes to women, by looking at what happens when females develop PCOS, we can see the role that androgens play in acne in both females and males.

PCOS

PCOS can be brought on by genetics or from disruptions in circadian rhythms. In Erica's case, the disruption in her circadian rhythm was the straw that broke the camel's back, causing disruption in her hormone balance. For some women, acne is the first noticeable signal they get that they are developing PCOS. (PCOS is commonly associated with acne.) The most obvious consequence of PCOS is enlarged ovaries that contain small follicles that look like cysts. Fortunately, these are not cancerous.

During their childbearing years, 7% to 10% of women have PCOS. In the US alone, according to the CDC, somewhere between 6% and 12% of reproductive-age women have PCOS, which is between five and six million women. It is the most common cause of infertility. Genetic predisposition definitely plays a role, but for others, PCOS can be induced by stress or disruption of the normal circadian rhythms—for example, some women can develop PCOS from working the night shift for an extended period of time. Most women who do have PCOS are not even aware that they have it. However, there are tests that show which hormones are imbalanced in the case of PCOS. Common imbalances occur in:

- → Estrogen
- → Progesterone
- → 17-OH Progesterone
- → LH/FSH ratio

Additionally, androgen excess is present in 60% to 80% of patients with PCOS. Elevated insulin levels can increase androgen levels, and abnormalities in how the brain or pituitary gland communicates with the ovaries may also lead to androgen overproduction. Other hormones from the ovaries or fat tissue may also be involved.

Over time, decreased sensitivity to insulin, obesity, sleep apnea, cardiac issues, and fatty liver are long-term side effects of PCOS. Moreover, the post adolescent and young female adult PCOS population will likely experience complications during pregnancy.

CONNECTIONS BETWEEN ACNE AND METABOLIC SYNDROME FOR MEN *AND* WOMEN

JAMA Dermatology reported in April of 2016 that post adolescent male patients with acne more commonly have insulin resistance and may be prediabetic, which are factors involved in metabolic syndrome. (Androgens are known to enlarge sebaceous glands, increase sebum production, and elevate keratin cells in the epidermis. *These three factors can cause acne.*) The same article also revealed that metabolic syndrome plays a key role in Polycystic Ovarian Syndrome. The effect of metabolic syndrome on PCOS shows up as:

→ Impaired hypothalamic-pituitary-adrenal axis
→ An increase in steroid hormones (steroidogenesis)
→ Insulin resistance
→ Abnormalities in the metabolic profile, e.g. a higher body mass index (BMI)

All of these set the stage for PCOS and are also factors in the development of acne in young male adults.

MAKING SURE YOUR HORMONES COOPERATE

Knowing how your hormones work together in balance is a little like walking a tightrope and holding a bar to keep yourself steady. In this case, the bar is the accumulation of everything you do to care for yourself and listen to your body. The bar represents becoming aware of the habits you need to stop *and* the habits you need to develop. I have faith that you will now take the following actions more seriously:

→ Doing proper and accurate hormone testing
→ Achieving the proper microbiome balance through diet and sometimes supplementation
→ Controlling your sugar intake
→ Establishing a fail-proof stress reduction routine

Once your maintenance routines shift, you will be able to walk the tightrope with ease.

Erica's Story, Continued

Remember Erica? She had been struggling with severe cystic acne ever since she had finished college and entered the workforce. By the time she came to see me, she felt like she was running out of options. The only thing left for her to try was Accutane, but because of its known side effects, she wasn't keen on that idea. We decided to do extensive testing to try and discover the root cause of her acne.

When I got the results of her hormone tests back, it was very clear that the pattern of her hormone imbalance fit the profile of Polycystic Ovarian Syndrome (PCOS). PCOS, also called Stein-Leventhal syndrome, occurs when a woman has abnormally high levels of androgen hormones. These hormones (testosterone, DHEA) are typically higher in males. Because PCOS is a syndrome, it is defined by a group of symptoms: acne, facial hair, anovulatory cycles, or amenorrhea (absence of menstrual cycles).

We started Erica on a tailored regimen to rebalance her hormones, remove the problematic microbes, and rebalance her microbiome. It definitely took of work, commitment, and patience on her part, but after six months of working to address her internal root causes, she noticed a significant change in her skin and was no longer developing new cysts.

CHAPTER SEVEN

THE FLAME IS INFLAMMATION

"Sebum is the fuel of the acne flame."

~PLEWIG AND KLIGMAN

I invite you to take this self-assessment quiz. Please answer either "yes" or "no" to the following:

- → Do you suffer from fatigue?
- → Do you have allergies?
- → Do you have gas, diarrhea, bloating, or constipation?
- → Does your skin have blotchy red areas?
- → Do you suffer from depression, anxiety, or brain fog?
- → Do you have headaches or migraines?
- → Do you have joint or muscle pain?
- → Do you struggle with your blood glucose levels?

Chronic inflammation can present itself in the body in a variety of ways. Acne, for example, is a systemic inflammatory condition.

DEFINING INFLAMMATION

All acne lesions are inflamed. Inflammation is what causes pores to become clogged to begin with and cause acne lesions to form.[9] Oily skin does not automatically cause acne—abnormal oil trapped within the pore is what causes the problem. Oil produced in response to inflammation is abnormal and has a thicker viscosity that is more likely to clog pores.

"Inflammation" is the broad term used to describe when your immune system gets fired up. It's a natural function with a bad reputation. Inflammation is not always a bad thing—in certain situations, we need our immune system to kick in to save our life. Without inflammation, injuries could fester and infections could become deadly. Although inflammation is a word that most of us associate with pain, discomfort, and poor health, it's intended to actually help us.

The problem comes when the inflammation is constant over a long period of time. This is how many medical conditions develop, because when there is a chronic low level of inflammation, chronic diseases occur.

When the body is injured, inflammation is a signal to the immune system to send white blood cells to the site of the injury so that the healing process can begin. (White blood cells produce inflammatory chemical mediators called cytokines.) Unfortunately, when inflammation goes on for too long, it can potentially trigger numerous other chronic health issues, including skin issues, fatigue, brain fog, depression, cancers, heart disease, arthritis, allergies, autoimmune conditions etc. Some say that inflammation is the "new cholesterol" due to its direct link to heart disease. In some cases, inflammation occurs when the immune

9 Perricone, *The Clear Skin Prescription*

system revolts against us and attacks our own bodies. This is what causes autoimmune diseases, including rheumatoid arthritis, type 1 diabetes, and IBD, among dozens of others. There are over 80 different autoimmune diseases.

WHAT CAUSES INFLAMMATION

Inflammation is a complex puzzle, but let's walk through some of the biggest triggers in acne sufferers based on what we understand in medicine and what I've seen clinically.

DIET

The diet the average American eats is highly inflammatory: it consists of grains, dairy, fried foods, foods full of sugar, and hidden sources of sugar.

Foods can cause inflammation by causing allergic responses, spiking blood sugar levels, causing leaky gut, increasing levels of arachidonic acid, and shifting the microbiome in a way that fuels bacterial overgrowth. Dietary choices can influence both the amount of sebum production and the composition of sebum.

High-glycemic-load foods like refined carbohydrates initiate an inflammatory cascade in the body and cause an unhealthy shift in the microbiome that results in an overgrowth of yeast and unfriendly bacteria.

Food Reactions

Food reactions can be broken down into two categories: food allergies and food sensitivities. Food *allergies* involve acute, immediate reactions to ingesting a food. After consuming a problematic food, most people with acute food allergies have a reaction from within minutes to up to three hours of consumption. Food *sensitivities* are delayed reactions to foods—it may take those reactions anywhere from 72 hours to three weeks after ingestion to emerge. In contrast to food allergies, food sensitivities can be much less obvious and much more difficult to identify because of the time lapse between ingesting the problematic food and experiencing a reaction.

Oftentimes, people are aware of the foods they're having immediate allergic reactions to because they notice the symptoms right away. However, even with allergies, there is a continuum, so a person could have an IgE (antibody) response that is less severe and not be aware of it. The most severe allergic reactions are life-threatening.

What Are Common Causes of Food Reactions?

Some of the most common contributing factors to food sensitivities are nutritional deficiencies, genetics, poor digestion, lack of variety in your diet, chronic infections, and intestinal hyper-permeability (also called leaky gut).

Most Common Food Allergies

- ➜ Gluten
- ➜ Dairy
- ➜ Eggs
- ➜ Fish
- ➜ Shellfish
- ➜ Tree Nuts
- ➜ Peanuts

➜ Soy

Symptoms That Can Be A Sign of Food Allergies

The following are vague symptoms that can be associated with food allergies. (This is not an exhaustive list.)

➜ Acne
➜ Skin rashes
➜ Brain fog
➜ Depression
➜ Headaches/migraines
➜ Sinus problems
➜ Indigestion/heartburn
➜ Joint pain
➜ Constipation/diarrhea
➜ Gas/bloating
➜ Weight retention
➜ Other skin problems

HOW GLUTEN IS CONNECTED TO DIGESTIVE ISSUES AND LEAKY GUT

Many people with acne have difficulty digesting gluten, meaning that it travels through their digestive system without being fully broken down. When this happens, it can cause damage to the delicate tissue that lines the intestines and thus cause a leaky gut. This in turn can trigger an immune response that can manifest as acne.

Contrary to mainstream information, gluten is not an individual protein found only in wheat, barley, and rye—it is a family of proteins that are found in all grains. Gluten is made of two types of proteins: prolamins and glutelins. All grains contain these prolamins and glutelins. While gliadin is a prolamin in wheat that has been studied extensively in medical research and gets a lot of attention, the prolamins in other grains can have a similar effect to gliadin in sensitive individuals. Prolamins are found in wheat, rye, and barley in higher percentages compared to some of the other grains, so this is possibly where the confusion comes in.

HOW DAIRY IS CONNECTED TO DIGESTIVE ISSUES AND LEAKY GUT

Dairy is another common reactionary food for acne sufferers. Although many people assume that dairy reactions trace back to lactose (the sugar found in milk), reactions can also be caused by the proteins in dairy. There are two types of protein found in dairy: whey and casein. Caseins are considered to be the more "allergenic" of the two proteins, which means that people more commonly have a sensitivity to casein. When casein is not fully broken down during digestion, it can damage the delicate tissue that lines the intestines and cause leaky gut. Again, this triggers inflammation that can fuel acne.

Another way that dairy can cause problems for acne sufferers is by stimulating a hormone called insulin-like growth factor or IGF-1. (IGF-1 promotes sebum production, and it's also the major growth hormone produced during puberty.)

Dairy consumption can disrupt hormone balance because of the hormones it contains. Organic milk may seem like a logical alternative, but it's important to understand that even organic milk is high still high in hormones because the cows that are used to produce milk are kept pregnant in order to keep them producing milk. Some of the hormones found in dairy products are prolactin, estrogens, progesterone, cortisol, and testosterone.

Dairy products promote a sluggish lymphatic system. This is why pretty much any detox program or detox diet will suggest eliminating dairy. However, a sluggish lymphatic system does not hinder strep from traveling—in fact, it's easier for strep to travel because all of your normal defense mechanisms (e.g., lymphocytes) are impaired.

In addition, some scientists believe that an acne-causing LPS-producing bacteria that we discussed earlier (i.e., pseudomonas) can cause people to be sensitive to dairy. Perhaps not surprisingly, many acne sufferers find relief by eliminating dairy from their diet.

BLOOD SUGAR ISSUES

Remember, acne is often referred to as "diabetes of the skin." Refined grains and other processed foods that are low in fiber have a higher glycemic load, meaning that they will spike blood sugar and trigger a process of inflammation that in some people can lead to acne breakouts.

That's because sugar consumption not only raises blood sugar, it also shifts the balance of the microbiome and tips it toward yeast and bacterial overgrowth. In contrast, complex carbohydrates are high in fiber. They feed good bacteria and help keep blood sugar stable. In the digestive health chapter, we talked about how bacteria and other microbes can cause acne. Well, that's for a simple reason: these organisms thrive on sugar.

STRESS

Stress-related changes to the composition of the microbiome can increase the likelihood and severity of intestinal permeability, which creates the perfect environment for systemic inflammation as well as local inflammation in the skin. In the chapter on hormone balance, we discussed how psychological stress triggers hormone balance and depresses our immune defenses. Psychological stress can actually set off a cascade of inflammatory chemicals! Stress leads to production of interleukin-1, an inflammatory cytokine that acts as a cellular messenger. When interleukin-1 levels are high, they can cause cells within the pore to become sticky and clog the pore, resulting in an acne lesion. Foods that are inflammatory can also increase production of interleukin-1.

PATHOGENS AND INFECTIONS

These disrupt the regular chain of events and the normal balance that is needed to maintain a healthy microbiome and healthy digestive function. When this happens, inflammation is a direct result. In the digestive health chapter, we talked about how some types of acne-causing bacteria produce a toxin called lipopolysaccharide or LPS. Poor digestion and consuming foods that are high in sugar (i.e., simple carbohydrates) promotes the overgrowth of LPS-producing bacteria. When leaky gut is present, LPS can reach high levels in the bloodstream and be highly inflammatory. This is referred to as metabolic endotoxemia, which is a driving force behind metabolic disease. LPS can also cause food allergies.

LEAKY GUT

Leaky gut is a condition wherein the barrier between your digestive tract and your bloodstream is compromised. When this happens, toxic byproducts of digestion that pass through your digestive tract (and normally stay within it) can cross over into your bloodstream and cause inflammation. Over time, your immune system can become overactive as a result of these byproducts being in the wrong place. This is one of the ways that autoimmune conditions can develop. Gluten is the most significant causative factor behind leaky gut in most people, but some other known causes are bacterial overgrowth, stress (psychological and physical), alcohol, pain medications, nutritional deficiencies, and environmental toxins.

NUTRITIONAL DEFICIENCIES

Each of these nutrients has known anti-inflammatory activities and is involved in neutralizing free radicals. They need to be kept at healthy levels to fight inflammation by preventing systemic inflammation:

- → Vitamin A
- → Vitamin B2
- → Vitamin B6
- → Vitamin C
- → Vitamin D
- → Vitamin E

➡ Selenium

➡ Zinc

➡ Omega-3 fatty acids

➡ CoQ10

➡ Glutamine

➡ Alpha Lipoic Acid

➡ Glutathione

➡ Magnesium

➡ Copper

HOW TO FIND OUT IF THE FOODS YOU'RE EATING ARE CAUSING INFLAMMATION

The most common way to identify foods that are causing inflammation is to do a food sensitivity blood test that looks for immune reactions to a predetermined list of 100 or more foods. The alternative to food sensitivity testing is to do a structured elimination/rotation diet where common food sensitivities are avoided for a period of 30 to 60 days, then reintroduced one at a time as you look out for any symptoms or reactions to them. Multiple food allergies are a symptom of a deeper problem.

All food sensitivity testing is not created equal. There are many food sensitivity tests that are easily available. You want a test that provides clinically valid results that are reproducible. To get access to professional grade food sensitivity testing we recommend, visit wellaheadchicago.com/shop?category=Testing

CHAPTER EIGHT

TAKING OUT THE GUESSWORK

"Do something today that your future self will thank you for."

~SEAN PATRICK FLANERY

In the previous chapters, you learned about underlying imbalances in the body that can trigger acne. In this chapter, you're going to learn how to test for all of the factors and root causes that influence the development of acne. People sometimes feel that it only makes sense to do laboratory tests if they have a medical condition that's more severe or is life-threatening. But here's the thing: *it's not just acne.* The same imbalances that cause acne can cause more serious and even life-threatening conditions. It's wise to take these imbalances seriously.

If you are someone who is *only experiencing acne breakouts* and nothing else right now, you're in a great position! You have a window of opportunity to get things under control and get healthier *before a more serious condition develops.*

SKIN FUNCTION

Many factors determine how severe acne breakouts are: how many strains of bacteria overgrowth you have, what the toxic load in your liver is, how many courses of antibiotics you have taken in your lifetime, what you eat, your hormone balance, etc.

THE SOLUTION

Step 1: Clean up your diet
Step 2: Get on a skin care regimen that's suited to your skin type
Step 3: Get on a basic supplement regimen
Step 4: Reduce your chemical exposure
Step 5: Take your regimen to the next level with helpful tests

The mistake that most people make is looking for a single natural remedy to cure their acne breakouts. Considering that acne is a complex condition that is caused by multiple factors, it makes sense that there isn't *one* supplement or natural remedy that is going to universally work for acne in every person. This is why it's really important to work with a holistic doctor who can help you identify the regimen that is right for you based on your root causes.

We've covered a lot of information about the internal root causes of acne! At this point, the natural question is "What can I do about it?" The easiest place to start is with *adjusting and cleaning up your diet and incorporating nutrient*-dense foods to foster a balanced microbiome, balanced hormones, and healthy liver function.

STEP 1: CLEAN UP YOUR DIET

"When you have acne, it's a misguided perception to think you can continue to eat junk food but use the right skin care products and have clear skin."

~DR. SHAYNA PETER

An anti-acne diet should be low in grains, refined sugars, alcohol, fried foods, and trans fats.

Any grain you eat should be in low in gluten and have a low glycemic load. Foods with a high glycemic load are converted quickly into sugar and spike insulin levels.

FOODS TO AVOID

Refined sugars

Reading labels and avoiding processed foods will help you reduce the amount of added sugar in your diet. Important note: Don't replace sugar with artificial sweeteners! They are not broken down in the digestive system and can accumulate in other parts of the body. Some healthier alternatives to sugars and artificial sweeteners are xylitol, monk fruit, and stevia. Natural sweeteners like coconut sugar, maple syrup, and honey should only be consumed in small amounts.

Refined carbohydrates and gluten

White rice, corn, processed potatoes, and products made with refined flour are all refined carbohydrates, meaning that they are low in fiber and will cause your blood sugar to rise rapidly.

When you eat carbohydrates, you want to make sure they are unrefined carbohydrates that are high in fiber, as this will keep them from spiking your blood sugar. There should be 3 grams of fiber for every 100 calories.

Gluten can be a trigger for many acne sufferers. All grains contain some form of gluten, so there are technically no "gluten-free" grains. Wheat and corn should definitely be avoided. Some people are able to still have grains like oats, rice, and quinoa and are still able to notice improvement in their acne.

> **Bonus Feature: To learn more about facts and myths about gluten, check out this video: https://blt.ly/3c1zLnl**

Dairy

We've discussed how dairy disrupts hormone balance and feeds bacteria, but dairy can also be a source of exposure to gluten—most cows are grain-fed, so milk and other by-products could still potentially have gluten. Also, there is cross-reactivity between gluten and dairy, so many people whose skin reacts to gluten also react to dairy.

Alcohol

Avoid consumption of alcohol. It puts undue stress on detoxifications systems, shifts the microbiome toward bacteria and yeast overgrowth, damages the intestinal lining, and raises blood sugar. According to the Global Burden of Diseases study, there is no safe amount of alcohol to consume.

Caffeine

Caffeine should be avoided. Long-term overconsumption of caffeine stresses the adrenal glands, heart, and thyroid glands, which is definitely counterproductive to healing acne. Caffeine can even exacerbate premenstrual syndrome (PMS). If you find that you need coffee in order to have energy, you owe it to yourself to find out the reason why.

Fried foods

Fried foods should be avoided and hydrogenated or trans fats should be avoided. These fats increase sebum production and also change the lipid ratio of sebum.

When choosing oils, it's best to stick with organic, cold-pressed oils. However, it's better to get your healthy fats from whole foods rather than oils—for example, eating olives instead of using olive oil or eating guacamole instead of using avocado oil. When cooking, use oils that are heat-stable and suited to the cooking temperature you're using. As an example, when foods are fried, they're generally cooked at higher temperatures, and many oils change their composition when heated at high temperatures. This how harmful byproducts and trans fats are formed. Oils and fats that are primarily made of saturated fats (coconut oil, palm oil, butter, ghee) are better-suited to high-heat cooking.

FOODS TO EAT

Choose grains that are low-glycemic and do not contain wheat. Some examples are brown rice, gluten-free oats, quinoa, and buckwheat. (Contrary to its name, buckwheat does not contain wheat.)

Helpful tip: Soak your grains and beans overnight before you cook them. This will reduce the amount of phytates, make them more digestible, and greatly shorten their cooking time also.

Eating Organic

Choose organic meats, preferably grass-fed, and choose eggs that are from pastured hens. whenever possible. Seafood should be wild-caught instead of farm-raised whenever possible. Because grass-fed animals and wild-caught seafood are fed a diet that is close to their natural diet, they have a healthier ratio of omega-6 to omega-3 fatty acids. In some stores, only responsibly farmed rather than wild-caught fish might be available. I would consider this to be a viable alternative. Responsibly farmed fish helps supplement the supply of wild-caught fish, which is low. Keep in mind that meat and seafood can be another potential source of antibiotics if they are not organic. We discussed in earlier chapters how antibiotics can disrupt the microbiome and stress the body's detoxification systems.

> **For suggestions on organic, grass-fed, and pasture raised meats, check out the resources section**

Vegetables and fruits

Eat your veggies! That's eight to ten half-cup servings daily. Choose a rainbow of colors—that way, you'll benefit from a wide variety of natural plant chemicals and antioxidants. A green powder from green veggies like spinach and broccoli can be a great addition, too. Eating lots of vegetables will give you plenty of fiber and prebiotics that will promote healthy bowel movements and feed good bacteria to restore and maintain a healthy microbiome.

Always choose organic produce over conventional produce whenever possible. Refer to the Environmental Working Group's "Dirty Dozen" and "Clean Fifteen" lists. These list the produce with the highest amounts of pesticides and the lowest amounts of pesticides respectively and are updated every year. But bear in mind that non-organic produce—even if low in pesticides or if you can peel away the skin—can still be genetically modified.

Water

I can't stress enough how important it is to drink water! The National Academies of Science, Engineering, and Medicine recommends that generally healthy women drink about 9 cups of water a day and generally healthy men drink about 12.5 cups a day. This does not include water intake from foods. Don't use thirst as your indicator, because by the time you're feeling thirsty, you're already dehydrated. Your urine should be light yellow in color. It's critical to drink purified water! We'll go into this further as we review ways to reduce our exposure to chemicals.

MEAL TIMING

Make sure there are 12 hours between your dinner and breakfast. This will help normalize your blood sugar response. In the evening, digestion slows down, so dinner should be your lightest meal of the day. Your last meal should be at least 2 hours before bedtime. These habits will promote complete digestion of your food.

MEAL PLANNING

Commit to planning your meals every week. It's easy to find yourself hungry while you're out and then to just reach for anything. Planning out your meals and packing your lunches will help you put thought into your food choices. It's a lot easier to stay out of the fast-food drive-thru when you have your meals planned out and you know what you're going to eat! Like the old adage says, "If you fail to plan, you plan to fail."

Check out the resource section at the very end of the book for meal-planning resources—you can choose from thousands of recipes that are adaptable to special diets.

TIPS FOR EATING OUT

If you know you're going out to eat, take a look at the menu beforehand so you already have an idea what the restaurant offers that falls within your regimen. (If the restaurant you're considering doesn't have those options, you can choose a different place to eat.) Many restaurants even provide calorie information. This will be especially helpful in spotting dishes that are too high in fat, which can be a problem for some acne sufferers. For example, you might automatically assume that a salad is the healthiest option...until you see its accompanying calorie information.

STEP 2: GET ON A SKIN CARE REGIMEN THAT'S SUITED TO YOUR SKIN TYPE

"Take care of your skin—it's going to be representing you for a long time."

~LINDEN TYLER

The long-term solution for acne goes deeper than skincare. However skincare is an important part of a comprehensive approach to acne. The best products for acne are going to be clean, hypoallergenic products that are suitable for your individual skin type. By "clean," I mean products made with the most natural ingredients that are free of chemicals that disrupt hormone balance. These days, we have to be very intentional when it comes to choosing products to use on our skin.

Don't automatically assume your skin is oily because you have acne—many acne sufferers actually do *not* have oily skin. For some, the oiliness of their skin is a rebound oil production from dry skin. Whether your skin is oily or not, you don't want to use products on your skin that are too harsh and overly drying. These are big mistakes that many people make when trying to heal their acne.

With acne, the skin barrier is compromised. It's extremely important that the skin care regimen you are following fights acne breakouts *and nourish*es the skin barrier, because that's what going to help your skin heal and reduce the inflammation.

Disruption of the skin barrier is part of how acne forms. The skin has three components: the epidermis, the dermis, and the hypodermis. The outermost layer of your epidermis is called the stratum corneum. This is also referred to as the skin barrier. When microbes from the digestive tract travel through the lymphatic system and enter the layers of the skin, they disrupt the skin barrier and cause blemishes. If you want to fight this process at the level of the skin, you have to strengthen the skin barrier.

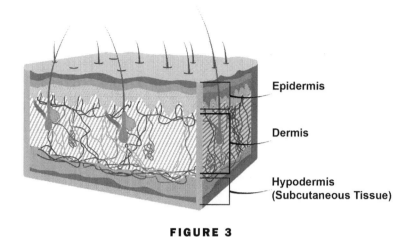

Epidermis

Dermis

Hypodermis
(Subcutaneous Tissue)

FIGURE 3

KNOW YOUR SKIN TYPE

It's also important to know your skin type. Believe it or not, one of the best ways to identify your skin type is to observe how your skin responds to products—observe which ones make them feel too oily or too dry and adjust accordingly. There are five main skin types:

→ Normal
→ Combination
→ Oily
→ Dry
→ Sensitive

> If you are unsure of your skin type, take this short quiz to find out: WellAheadChicago.com/skincare

FIGURE OUT YOUR SKIN CARE REGIMEN

Your skin care regimen should consist of these basic components at a minimum:

- → Cleanser
- → Toner
- → Moisturizer
- → Sunscreen
- → Exfoliant
- → Spot treatment
- → Optional: dark spot treatment

Your cleanser, toner, and moisturizer should suited to your skin type. All skin care products you use should be as natural as possible and gentle on your skin.

Cleanser

Many commercial cleansers are available. If you wear makeup, you should double-cleanse when removing your makeup. This will help give your skin a good cleaning without stripping your skin of its oils and overly drying your skin.

How to double-cleanse: first cleanse your skin with an oil- or cream-based cleanser in order to remove your makeup, then cleanse your skin with a foam- or gel-based cleanser that works into a lather to thoroughly cleanse your skin once the makeup has been removed.

Toner

There are different schools of thought on toner. Some skin experts say that toner is not necessary if your cleanser is effective while others say that toners should be used to remove excess oil from the skin. Your toner should restore your skin pH and prep your skin for the next step in your routine. When choosing a toner, you want a formula that is not overly drying. (That has to do with how it's applied to your skin and what's in the formula itself.)

Moisturizer

Whether your skin is normal, dry, oily, combination, or sensitive, you still need to moisturize. Your moisturizer should be suited for your skin type to maintain the proper oil balance and nourish your skin barrier.

Sunscreen

Sunscreen is going to be especially important while going through the healing process because some exfoliating and acne-fighting ingredients can make skin more sensitive to sun exposure. Dark marks from acne can also be worsened by sun exposure. In addition to sunscreen, consuming plenty of antioxidants in your daily meals or even taking them in supplement form will also help to protect your skin from discoloration caused by sun exposure. Keep in mind that sun exposure has positive health benefits as well, such as vitamin D production (which helps control acne) and melatonin production (a hormone that regulates the sleep cycle).

When choosing sunscreens, look for cream/lotion formulas that contain physical blockers instead of chemical blockers. Some examples of physical blockers are titanium dioxide and zinc oxide; some common chemical blockers are oxybenzone and octinoxate, which are known endocrine disruptors. Avoid sprays and powders. If you're looking for cream-based sunscreen formulas with physical blockers that don't leave a chalky white residue behind, check out the resources section at the end of the book.

Exfoliant

Chemical exfoliants like alpha and beta hydroxy acids can be very helpful for acne-prone skin—they help promote smooth skin texture by breaking down healed lesions and lightening dark marks. Using these once or twice per week can make a dramatic difference. Before applying them to your face, however, you should always test a patch of skin in an area that is not exposed and observe your reaction.

Spot Treatment

Having a good spot treatment on hand can help minimize the damage to your complexion from acne breakouts by helping breakouts to heal faster, reducing scarring and dark marks.

Below are examples of acne-fighting ingredients that may be found in natural, non-irritating acne spot treatments:

- White willow bark
- Benzyl peroxide
- Salicylic acid
- Lactic acid
- Spearmint oil
- Tea tree oil
- Saw palmetto
- Resorcinol monoacetate
- Neem oil
- Menthol
- Sulfur
- Coconut oil

Dark Spot Treatment

Post-acne hyperpigmentation is the technical term for excess pigment in the skin. Dark marks left behind after an acne breakout has healed are often a very distressing issue for acne sufferers, because they can take several months to fade and they become particularly problematic when people have recurring breakouts in the same area. Both exfoliants and dark spot treatments can lighten dark marks from acne. Dark marks from acne can be worsened by sun exposure, so sun protection is very important, whether it's in the form of a topical sunscreen or an antioxidant supplement.

Below are key ingredients often used in natural skin care formulas for dark spots:

→ Arbutin
→ Vitamin C
→ Pycnogenol
→ Licorice extract
→ Kojic acid

Skin of color is more susceptible to hyperpigmentation. Hydroquinone has been considered for many years and the gold standard for treating hyperpigmentation in both OTC and prescription products. Many people have concerns about using hydroquinone on their skin over an extended period of time or using it on their skin at all. These are very valid concerns. Hydroquinone is considered one of the top seven cancer-causing ingredients in personal care products, and it has been banned in the European Union and many other countries around the world. However, hydroquinone continues to be approved by the U.S. Food and Drug Administration despite health concerns because it's used in lower concentrations and it's used on smaller areas of the skin compared to how it was previously used in other countries. That said, as you are becoming more aware of the chemicals you are exposed to on a daily basis from a variety of sources, it is definitely reasonable to look for alternatives that are less toxic such as our Brightening Vitamin C Serum (wellaheadchicago. com/shop/vitamin-c-serum).

> **For a simple acne-fighting, natural skincare regimens for all skin types, visit:**
> **www.DrShaynaPeter.com/Quickstart**

STEP 3: GET ON A BASIC SUPPLEMENT REGIMEN

Just eating healthy is not enough these days—the air is polluted, the soil is depleted of nutrients, the water is polluted. Produce loses nutrient content as it travels long distances to reach a store and then as it sits on a shelf. Even if we're on our best dining behavior, most of us are still going to have deficiencies if we are relying on diet alone to maintain our health. It's just the world we live in. You've got to supplement your healthy lifestyle!

In Chapter Three, we went over the vitamins and minerals that play important roles in skin health and that are commonly deficient in people who have persistent acne. A supplement regimen for acne sufferers would include these nutrients but would also be personalized by doing advanced testing to uncover deficiencies and help determine what form of the supplement to take, what amount of it, and for what period of time.

Omega-3 fatty acids are essential for most people who follow a standard American diet. Unless we're making an additional effort, most of us are eating diets that are deficient in omega-3 fatty acids (which are anti-inflammatory) and very high in omega-6 fatty acids (which are pro-inflammatory). When supplementing with omega-3s, it's really important to take a high-quality formula that is highly bioavailable and has been purified to remove mercury.

High-quality multivitamins are important for acne sufferers. These should contain highly absorbable versions of nutrients that are commonly deficient in acne sufferers that we've discussed in previous chapters. They should also contain therapeutic levels like our Clear Well Multi (wellaheadchicago. com/shop/clear-well-multi).

Digestive enzymes can provide essential digestive support to make sure carbohydrates, proteins, and fats are being fully broken down so they are not causing inflammation and feeding bad bacteria. Digestion is often diminished in acne sufferers, especially if bacteria or fungal overgrowth is present.

Probiotics help restore healthy levels of good bacteria and maintain the integrity of the intestinal barrier. Their presence out-competes pathogens and inhibits their overgrowth. Probiotics also support vaginal health in women. **Prebiotics** help feed good bacteria. The availability of probiotic strains on the market is limited. There are numerous probiotic strains present in our microbiome that are not available on the market in a probiotic form, so taking prebiotics is the only way to increase them.

Vitamin D deficiency is often the reason why people have more acne flares in the wintertime—remember, sunlight is our main source of vitamin D—and most multivitamins do not contain adequate levels of vitamin D.

B-complex deficiencies are common in acne sufferers. B vitamins work synergistically, so it's always best to take them in the form of a complex. If you have had all your B vitamin levels tested and know for sure that you are deficient in a specific vitamin, then it makes sense to take more of that specific vitamin in addition to a B complex.

Zinc deficiency is also common among acne sufferers, but it's important to take zinc in the form of a multi-vitamin/ multi-mineral formula with the proper zinc-to-copper ratio *unless* a deficiency has been identified with lab testing. Clear Well Multi has therapeutic levels of zinc, B-vitamins, vitamin D, and other key nutrients (discussed in Chapter Three) that support clear, radiant skin. (Learn more at: wellaheadchicago.com/shop/clear-well-multi).

DO YOUR SUPPLEMENT RESEARCH

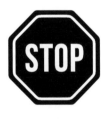

Caution!

Beware of purchasing supplements in drugstores! They are not the same quality as professional-grade supplements. Numerous exposés have showed that drugstore supplements do not contain the advertised amounts of the ingredients on the label. Many people whom I've tested had been taking drugstore vitamins for years and they were still deficient in the nutrients they were supposedly taking.

> **If you want to know what products I recommend, here's a list of the of best products with the ingredients I'm mentioning here in this chapter.**
> WellAheadChicago.com/blog/radiant

SUPPLEMENT ACTION STEPS

1. Make sure you are taking high-quality supplements that meet FDA standards. For physician-formulated product suggestions, visit: WellAheadChicago.com/blog/radiant

2. You can find more product suggestions along with instruction guides, example daily regimens, and more in my Clear Skin Quickstart Guide. To get your copy, visit: www.DrShaynaPeter.com/Quickstart

3. Go through your supplement regimen with your doctor to make sure you are taking the supplements that are appropriate for you.

STEP 4: REDUCE YOUR CHEMICAL EXPOSURE

Some of our biggest sources of exposure to chemicals are in:

→ Air
→ Water
→ Food
→ Personal care products
→ Plastic
→ Cleaning products

CHEMICALS ARE EVERYWHERE, SO WHAT'S THE BIG DEAL?

Excessive chemical exposure has been linked to health problems far more concerning than acne: autoimmune disease, cancer, heart disease, you name it. And yes, it can have an effect on acne, too. The problem with a lot of these chemicals is that when they get inside the body and into the bloodstream, they can mimic hormones. In an earlier chapter, we talked about how hormone imbalance affects acne. Well, many of these chemicals disrupt hormones, which is why they are referred to as xenohormones and endocrine disruptors. Xenohormones are chemicals made outside of the human body that have hormone-like effects in the body. Bear in mind that when it comes to insecticides and pesticides, even if they're banned in the US, they may still be used in other countries and we still may come across them when foods are imported. Also, chemicals can persist in the environment and in our food chain long after they have been banned. Here are some common endocrine disruptors (please note this not an exhaustive list):

Chemical Family	What it's used for	How you get exposed	How to reduce your exposure
Aluminum and metals		Deodorants, antiperspirants, food additives, non-stick teflon cookware, beverage bottles, metal food cans, lipsticks and eye makeup	Read labels to identify aluminum-based additives and consider alternatives.
Arsenic		Rice and rice-based products	Vary your grains. Cook rice like pasta: with an abundance of water. Rinse your rice.

Bisphenol (BPA, BPS)	Plasticizer	Lining of metal food and drink cans, plastic baby bottles and containers, hard plastic water bottles, paints, adhesives, enamels	Use BPA-free products. Reduce your use of canned foods; choose fresh foods. Never microwave food in plastic storage containers or plastic wrap!
Butylated hydroxyanisole (BHA)	Preservative	Chips and preserved meats	Check food labels and choose organic products.
Glycol ethers (PEG, Polyethylene glycols)	Solvent	Cosmetics, shampoos, personal cleaning products, solvents in paints, cleaning products, brake fluid	Check cosmetic and toiletry labels and reduce occupational exposure.
Lead		Paint, household dust, water pipes, imported canned food and imported hard candies, toys, pottery ceramics, batteries, color additives, lipsticks, eye makeups containing kohl	Filter your water and check labels of cosmetics, especially lipsticks. Use certified organic lip balm.
Oxybenzone and Octinoxate	UVB sunscreen	Chemical sunscreens	Choose a mineral-based sunscreen with zinc oxide and/or titanium dioxide as the active ingredients.
Mercury		Shellfish and fish, coal	Eat seafood that is low in mercury. Avoid canned fish products.
Methylisothiazolinone (named allergen of the year by The American Contact Dermatitis Society in 2013)		Personal care products, hair care products, pet products, yard care products	

Organophosphates	Pesticide	Apples, peaches, pears, plums, cherries, cotton, corn, wheat, nuts, cabbage, hops, lentils, oats, onions, rice, soybeans, beets, sunflowers	Buy organic produce.
Parabens (methylparaben, propylparaben, butylparaben etc.)	Preservative	Used in toiletries and personal care products: shampoos and conditioners, makeup, moisturizers, shaving products, and others	Check cosmetic and toiletry labels.
Perfluorinated chemicals	Teflon chemical	Food wrappers, carpet stain protectors, popular raincoats, Teflon pans	Skip non-stick pans as well as stain- and water-resistant coatings on clothing, furniture, and carpets.
Petrolatum, petroleum, mineral oil (polycyclic aromatic hydrocarbons and glycol ethers are petroleum byproducts)	Emollient, shine	Personal care products, cosmetics, baby lotions, cold creams, ointments, cosmetics	Use products that contain USP grade petroleum.
Phthalates ("Fragrance," "Parfum")	Plasticizer	Cosmetics, perfumes, candles, children's toys, food products, pharmaceuticals, syringes, blood bags and tubing (IV tubings, catheters, etc.)	Avoid containers, toys, and wraps made from PVC; avoid products that simply list "fragrance."
Triclosan	Antibacterial chemical	Liquid soaps, detergents, and other sanitizing products; toothpaste and hair products	Check ingredient labels.
Talc	Preservative	Cosmetics, aerosol sprays, chewing gum, supplements	Check ingredient labels.

HOW TO REDUCE DAILY EXPOSURE TO CHEMICALS

To reduce your chemical exposure, you're going to have to read labels a lot more carefully and become a lot more educated.

Personal Care Products

Personal care products are a way that chemicals can sneak into our body. The skin barrier looks strong, but actually many substances can cross over into our bloodstream through our skin—in fact, a number of formulas for hormone replacement are actually in the form of a skin cream. Other products contain chemicals that act like hormones (i.e., estrogen, progesterone, thyroid hormones, testosterone) when absorbed into your system and/or they can actually interfere with those hormones. This means that such products can contribute to acne. Another concern with synthetic chemicals is they can be harsh and damaging to the skin, which is definitely counterproductive when working to heal acne. Dealing with acne can be a vicious cycle if you're not careful!

Chemicals in Personal Care Products

Thousands of ingredients used in cosmetics, toiletries, candles, and cleaning products are disguised as "fragrance" or "parfum." These terms are able to legally hide numerous chemicals because they are treated as trade secrets.

AIR QUALITY

Air is one of the major ways that we're exposed to toxins in our everyday environments. Some sources are traffic pollution, mold, off-gassing from furniture and carpeting, paints, cleaning products, and nail polish. While we don't have as much control over traffic pollution, we do have some control of other factors, namely indoor air pollution. Indoor pollution is just as big of a problem as outdoor pollution! If you see mold spots in your home or believe there has been water damage, test your home with an ERMI kit.

SMOKING AND SECOND-HAND SMOKE

Most people are aware that smoking has been linked to numerous health problems for individuals who smoke, but cigarette smoke compromises the air quality in homes and impacts other members of the household who *don't* smoke, too. Additionally, smoking produces inflammation and free radicals and depletes the body's store of protective antioxidants.

WATER QUALITY

Filtering your water is a must! Tap water is not an option, especially given the fact that in some cities, up to 42 different prescription drugs have been found in the drinking water. There are a variety of water filters available on the market with varying levels of filtration depending on the price point.

Check out the resources section for more information on water filters and how to choose the right one for you.

OTHER LIFESTYLE STRATEGIES

Exercise

Get a move on! Commit to exercising regularly for a minimum of 30 to 45 minutes three to four times per week. Rebounding exercises like running, jumping jacks, and elliptical machines stimulate blood flow and promote healthy digestion and the flow of your lymphatic system, which filters waste in the body. Remember, the skin is the last organ to receive nutrients! Stimulating blood flow helps promote the delivery of nutrients to your skin. It's important to choose activities you enjoy.

Sleep

Sleep is a critical repair process in the body. You've got to get adequate sleep, which is a minimum of seven to eight hours per night. In research studies, just one night of sleep deprivation has been shown to spike cortisol levels. Sleep deprivation also leads to diminished immune function. In addition, poor sleep increases cravings by shifting the balance of satiety hormones. This can lead to poor food choices, and as we've previously discussed, high-calorie junk foods do not support a healthy microbiome. An unbalanced microbiome leads to other health problems.

Sleep is a must for overall health, healing, and hormone balance, so get your restorative beauty sleep every single night! Your sleep pattern should correspond with the sunrise and the sunset wherever you are in the world. If you are having difficulty falling asleep or are unable to sleep continuously throughout the night, work with your doctor to figure out why.

RECAPPING YOUR LIFESTYLE STRATEGIES

Honing these key lifestyle tips will get you off to a great start

1. Maintain a healthy diet
2. Reduce your chemical exposure
3. Stay hydrated
4. Get good sleep
5. Reduce your stress
6. Supplement your healthy lifestyle

In the resources section, you'll find products that will help you reduce your chemical exposure.

STEP 5: TAKE YOUR REGIMEN TO THE NEXT LEVEL WITH HELPFUL TESTS

THE SICK CARE MODEL

One of the biggest mistakes people make when it comes to their health is thinking that they have health care. We do not have a health care system. We have a disease management system. Our health care model in the United States is intended for disease management, not wellness.

When you don't eat well and you don't exercise, when you smoke and drink too much alcohol, you put yourself into a compromised position, a position where eventually you will have medical problems and will need to take medications in order to function. When you're unwilling to do anything for your health unless your insurance covers it, you allow an insurance company to become your doctor and dictate your care instead of you and your doctor being in charge of your care.

If a doctor is not able to document that higher-level testing is medically necessary based on your medical history and your complaints, your insurance plan is unlikely to cover additional testing even if the tests will likely give both you and your doctor better direction for your care. Many people struggle with acne and health problems for years because their insurance will not cover the tests needed to properly diagnose their symptoms because they are not deemed medically necessary. It's worth setting aside a health budget and/or a flexible spending account for wellness services.

THE LIMITATIONS OF STANDARD LAB TESTS

After having a round of tests at their annual checkup, people are often told that everything is "normal." You might now be wondering how are functional lab tests different from tests that your primary doctor does—why isn't "normal" good enough? There are three main ways that standard lab tests are different from functional lab tests.

The Tests Themselves

Whether they are primary care providers or specialists, conventional doctors are not able to run enough tests to give a complete picture of your health and nutritional status because the tests they run are controlled by insurance. A patient has to have a specific set of symptoms in order for a doctor to justify running tests and have those tests be covered by insurance. Many tests that are done for wellness and to determine a person's health status when they *don't meet* specific diagnostic criteria are not considered medically necessary by insurance companies.

The Time Period the Tests Reflect

There are functional lab tests available that measure the levels of vitamins within the lymphocytes, a type of white blood cell. In comparison, standard conventional labs measure vitamin levels in the serum. Serum levels reflect only the snapshot in time when you had your blood drawn, whereas measuring the levels within lymphocytes provides a reflection of the last four to six months. (Lymphocytes have a lifecycle of four to six months.) That's a much more accurate reading. Serum tests can still be useful—in fact, it can be helpful to compare cellular levels of vitamins and minerals to serum levels of vitamins and minerals—but those two tests are measuring two different things.

The Grey Area

Standard lab tests often miss people who are in the "grey" area, that is, the people who have symptoms but do not fit a textbook diagnosis. Health is a continuum. For many people, acne is one of several symptoms they're experiencing. Their symptoms don't add up to a diagnosis, but they know something is off. Functional nutritional tests can be immensely helpful to people in these situations. Many tests and procedures produce false negatives because they are unable to identify low-grade problems—they only identify the problem if it's severe.

Reference Ranges

Another limitation with conventional testing is that in conventional settings, they are interpreted within a very wide reference range. But just because a lab result is within the reference range, that does not mean it's within the ideal range for that specific person. It is necessary to view these tests through a different lens. Let's use the example of thyroid hormones. Say a person has a "normal" level of thyroid-stimulating hormone (TSH). If you think of TSH like a shoe, size 6 and size 11 are both "normal" shoe sizes, but if neither of those sizes are not right for your foot, you're going to have a problem. It's the same thing with TSH. If a person's TSH is not at the optimal level for their body, they may very well have symptoms even though their level is technically within the normal range.

IMPORTANT TESTS

→ **Complete blood count** can be an important screening tool to achieve optimal immune function and decrease chronic infections in acne sufferers.

→ **Tests for micronutrients** (vitamins, minerals, etc.) measure your levels of 35 vitamins and minerals and omega fatty acids in your white blood cells. Vitamin and mineral analysis can reveal a person's functional nutrient status over a much longer time period than conventional serum testing does. This form of testing gives a more meaningful measurement of your nutritional status. Knowing your intracellular micronutrient levels is key to understanding your nutritional requirements. To access professional grade specialty testing we recommend, visit wellahead-chicago.com/shop/micronutrient-testing.

→ **Omega-3 index testing** measures your essential fatty acid ratio of omega-3s to omega-6s.

→ **Stool pathogen testing** detects the presence of the most common parasites or bacterial infections, viruses, and fungi, all of which affect digestive function, gut inflammation, and more. Measuring these factors is essential to assessing digestive health and knowing which steps to take in order to restore optimal digestive health.

→ **Lipopolysaccharide (LPS) testing** measures the levels of this inflammation-causing toxin produced by certain bacterial strains. This can help determine whether leaky gut is present.

→ **Cortisol and DHEA saliva testing** can give great insight into adrenal health, hormone balance, and the health of the body's fight-or-flight response.

→ **Sex hormone testing** measures the levels of estrogen, progesterone, and testosterone. Having a proper balance of these hormones is key in controlling breakouts. Often, when exposure to hormone-mimicking chemicals from toxins in foods and the environment are reduced, these hormones are able to balance out on their own without hormone replacement or other medications.

→ **Thyroid function testing** is critical. It is very important that thyroid hormone levels are not just within the reference range! At the very least, your TSH T3 and T4 should be checked, not just your TSH alone. There is a narrow range for optimal thyroid function.

→ **Blood sugar control tests** include fasting blood glucose, hemoglobin A1c, and insulin tests. These markers give key insights into blood sugar regulation, which is a key factor in fueling hormone imbalances, inflammation, imbalanced gut flora, etc.

→ **High-sensitivity C-reactive protein tests** measure systemic inflammation and repair.

TESTING FOR FOOD SENSITIVITIES/INTOLERANCES

We've discussed how foods high in sugar, gluten, and dairy can trigger acne. Testing to see if your body is producing an immune response to specific foods is a smart move—it will take out the guesswork about how your diet is affecting your skin. Lots of different types of food allergy tests are available. What I would recommend doing first is finding out if you are reacting to gluten and whether or not you have a leaky gut. This is done by a blood test that checks for antibodies to various forms of gluten.

If you do have a leaky gut, you're more likely to have multiple food sensitivities, and you will need to heal your gut in order to recover from some of those food sensitivities. But remember, there are several pieces to healing the gut: balancing hormones, supporting digestion, rebalancing the microbiome, correcting nutrient deficiencies, etc.

ACTION STEPS FOR TESTING

1. Take advantage of 21st century laboratory tests that can give you the insights you've been looking for! We're at a point in time where we have incredible technology that removes the guesswork. If you'd like to learn even more and access recommended specialty lab tests, check out our Clear Skin Accelerator Program at: https://www.drshaynapeter.com/accelerator

2. Work with your health care team to develop a short-term and a long term plan to get your health and lab results back to normal. If you are ready for professional analysis and guidance in optimizing skin health and full body wellness, you can learn more about our virtual health consulting programs at WellAheadChicago.com/natural-skincare

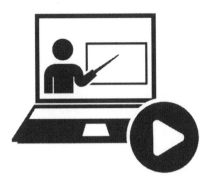

CONTINUING EDUCATION
FOR CLEAR SKIN

I love to keep up with the latest studies and research, and you can, too! Sign up for my newsletter at [bit.ly/drshaynanewsletter] to hear about the most recent scientific findings in the ever-evolving field of dermatology. In the meantime, if you want to accelerate your results even more with step-by-step video training and implementation guides, check out my Clear Skin Accelerator Program.

Learn more at www.DrShaynaPeter.com/Accelerator or connect with me on Instagram @drshaynaepeter. If you'd like to let other readers know about this book, you can leave a review at bit.ly/acnebookreview

MEET DR. SHAYNA E. PETER

MY STORY AND WHY I DO WHAT I DO

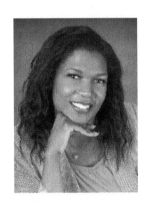

While I was completing my MD training and pursuing dermatology as a career, I began to struggle with acne for the first time in my life. After trying many different skin care products, antibiotics, topical medications, and aesthetic treatments, I had the experience of conventional treatment methods failing me as a patient. Most of the recommended treatments irritated my skin, made my skin very dry, and did not provide any lasting relief. Underneath it all, I knew there had to be a deeper root cause that was being ignored.

As a medical student rotating in dermatology, I saw many patients with severe autoimmune skin conditions. I was devastated by the limited treatment options that were available to them because many had very harmful adverse effects—I witnessed the damaging side effects of many of the harsh medications used to treat autoimmune conditions. As a doctor, I wanted to truly be able to "do no harm" and offer my patients safer treatment options that would also address the root causes of their skin conditions. My experiences are what led me to functional medicine and continue to fuel my passion and commitment to helping people with complex skin conditions and autoimmune disorders.

EDUCATION AND TRAINING

Dr. Shayna Peter is a Functional Medicine Naturopathic Doctor and Licensed Dietitian Nutritionist. Dr. Peter's unique blend of conventional MD training, naturopathic medicine training (NMD), and 13 years of experience in nutrition allows her to incorporate the best treatments that Eastern and Western medicine have to offer. Dr. Peter is also a published author in the Journal of American Academy of Dermatology and serves as an expert contributor on functional medicine and holistic dermatology to local and national media outlets.

Dr. Peter is a Chicago native. She completed her undergraduate studies at University of Illinois Urbana-Champaign in the College of Agricultural, Consumer, and Environmental Sciences, where she earned a Bachelor of Science in Nutrition with honors. She went on to work in the nonprofit sector, developing health programming for Chicago Public Schools. She also speaks Spanish and conversational Portuguese.

Dr. Peter completed her Doctor of Naturopathic Medicine through Meharry Medical College and the National University of Health Sciences. She believes that an integrative approach to health care is critically important and allows health providers to partner with individuals to explore treatment options that will provide the best outcomes while minimizing adverse effects.

Dr. Peter loves to keep up with the latest information and also help her community stay informed. In that spirit, she offers a newsletter highlighting the most recent advancements in holistic dermatology science. You can sign up for her free newsletter at [bit.ly/drshaynanewsletter], and you can connect with her on Instagram @drshaynaepeter.

REFERENCES

CHAPTER 2 | IT'S NOT JUST ACNE

1. Wang, S., 2005. Effects of psychological stress on small intestinal motility and bacteria and mucosa in mice. World Journal of Gastroenterology, [online] 11(13), p.2016. Available at: <https://www.ncbi.nlm.nih.gov/pmc/articles/PMC4305729/>.

2. Ketron, Lloyd W. "Gastro-intestinal Findings In Acne Vulgaris". *Journal Of The American Medical Association* no. 9 (1916): 671. doi:10.1001/jama.1916.02590090025008.

3. Volkova LA, Khalif IL, Kabanova[L1] IN: "Impact of the impaired intestinal microflora on the course of acne vulgaris". Klin Med (Mosk) 2001, 79:39-41, Russian.

4. Teitelman, G., T.H. Joh, and D.J. Reis. "Linkage Of The Brain-Skin-Gut Axis: Islet Cells Originate From Dopaminergic Precursors". *Peptides* 2 (1981): 157-168.

5. Burcelin R: Intestinal microflora, inflammation, and metabolic diseases. Abstract 019, Keystone Symposia - Diabetes Whistler, British Columbia, Canada; 2010.

6. Zhang, M., Qureshi, A. A., Fortner, R. T., Hankinson, S. E., Wei, Q., Wang, L. E., Eliassen, A. H., Willett, W. C., Hunter, D. J., & Han, J. (2015). Teenage acne and cancer risk in US women: A prospective cohort study. *Cancer, 121*(10), 1681–1687. https://doi.org/10.1002/cncr.29216

7. Danby, William. 2009. "Acne, Dairy And Cancer". *Dermato-Endocrinology 1* (1): 12-16. doi:10.4161/derm.1.1.7124.

8. Parida, Sheetal, and Dipali Sharma. 2019. "The Microbiome–Estrogen Connection And Breast Cancer Risk". *Cells* 8 (12): 1642. doi:10.3390/cells8121642.

9. Velicer, Christine M. 2004. "Antibiotic Use In Relation To The Risk Of Breast Cancer". JAMA 291 (7): 827. doi:10.1001/jama.291.7.827.

CHAPTER 3 | NUTRITIONAL DEFICIENCIES

1. Nakatsuji, Teruaki, Mandy C. Kao, Liangfang Zhang, Christos C. Zouboulis, Richard L. Gallo, and Chun-Ming Huang. "Sebum Free Fatty Acids Enhance The Innate Immune Defense Of Human Sebocytes By Upregulating -Defensin-2 Expression". *Journal Of Investigative Dermatology* 130, no. 4 (2010): 985-994. doi:10.1038/jid.2009.384.

2. Keen, MohammadAbid, and Iffat Hassan. "Vitamin E In Dermatology". *Indian Dermatology Online Journal* 7, no. 4 (2016): 311. doi:10.4103/2229-5178.185494.

3. Kucharska, Alicja, Agnieszka Szmurło, and Beata Sińska. "Significance Of Diet In Treated And Untreated Acne Vulgaris". *Advances In Dermatology And Allergology* 2 (2016): 81-86. doi:10.5114/ada.2016.59146.

4. National Institutes of Health. 2020. *Vitamin And Mineral Supplement Fact Sheets*. [online] Available at: <Ods. od.nih.gov. 2020. [online] Available at: <https://ods. od.nih.gov/factsheets/list-VitaminsMinerals/> [Accessed 9 July 2020].> [Accessed 22 February 2020].

5. Stough, Con, Tamara Simpson, Justine Lomas, Grace McPhee, Clare Billings, Stephen Myers, Chris Oliver, and Luke A Downey. "Reducing Occupational Stress With A B-Vitamin Focussed Intervention: A Randomized Clinical Trial: Study Protocol". *Nutrition Journal* 13, no. 1 (2014). doi:10.1186/1475-2891-13-122.

6. Rembe, Julian-Dario, Carolin Fromm-Dornieden, and Ewa Klara Stuermer. "Effects Of Vitamin B Complex And Vitamin C On Human Skin Cells". *Advances In Skin & Wound Care* 31, no. 5 (2018): 225-233. doi:10.1097/01.asw.0000531351.85866.d9.

7. Cspinet.org. 2020. *10 Worst Foods | Center For Science In The Public Interest*. [online] Available at: <https://cspinet.org/eating-healthy/foods-to-avoid/10-worst-foods> [Accessed 21 February 2020].

CHAPTER 4 | DIGESTIVE HEALTH
- GO WITH YOUR GUT

1. Maes, Michael, Ivana Mihaylova, and Jean-Claude Leunis. "Increased Serum Iga And Igm Against LPS Of Enterobacteria In Chronic Fatigue Syndrome (CFS): Indication For The Involvement Of Gram-Negative Enterobacteria In The Etiology Of CFS And For The Presence Of An Increased Gut–Intestinal Permeability". *Journal Of Affective Disorders* 99, no. 1-3 (2007): 237-240. doi:10.1016/j.jad.2006.08.021.

2. Bowe, Whitney P, and Alan C Logan. "Acne Vulgaris, Probiotics And The Gut-Brain-Skin Axis - Back To The Future?". *Gut Pathogens* 3, no. 1 (2011): 1. doi:10.1186/1757-4749-3-1.

3. Omran, AyatollahNasrollahi, and AlinaghiGhiasi Mansori. "Pathogenic Yeasts Recovered From Acne Vulgaris: Molecular Characterization And Antifungal Susceptibility Pattern". *Indian Journal Of Dermatology* 63, no. 5 (2018): 386. doi:10.4103/ijd.ijd_351_17..

4. Chassaing, Benoit, Lucie Etienne-Mesmin, and Andrew T. Gewirtz. "Microbiota-Liver Axis In Hepatic Disease". *Hepatology* 59, no. 1 (2013): 328-339. doi:10.1002/hep.26494.

CHAPTER 5 | LIVER FUNCTION - DETOXIFICATION

1. Simbrunner, Benedikt, Mattias Mandorfer, Michael Trauner, and Thomas Reiberger. "Gut-Liver Axis Signal-

ing In Portal Hypertension". *World Journal Of Gastroenterology* 25, no. 39 (2019): 5897-5917. doi:10.3748/wjg.v25.i39.5897.

2. "Dirty Dozen Endocrine Disruptors". EWG, 2020. https://www.ewg.org/research/dirty-dozen-list-endocrine-disruptors. Available at: <https://www.ewg.org/research/dirty-dozen-list-endocrine-disruptors> [Accessed 3 March 2020].

3. Margolis, David. "Acne And Group A Strep: An Unknown Burden". Grantome, 2020. Available at: http://grantome.com/grant/NIH/RO1-AR051185-03. [Accessed 3 March 2020].

4. American, S., 2020. *Why Are Trace Chemicals Showing Up In Umbilical Cord Blood?*. [online] Scientific American. Available at: <https://www.scientificamerican.com/article/chemicals-umbilical-cord-blood/> [Accessed 15 July 2020].

5. Analytical Services, A. and Research Ltd, F., 2005. *Body Burden: The Pollution In Newborns*. [online] EWG. Available at: <https://www.ewg.org/research/body-burden-pollution-newborns> [Accessed 15 July 2020].

6. William, A., 2018. *Medical Medium Liver Rescue: Answers To Eczema, Psoriasis, Diabetes, Strep, Acne, Gout, Bloating, Gallstones, Adrenal Stress, Fatigue, Fatty Liver, Weight Issues, SIBO & Autoimmune Disease*. Carlsbad: Hay House Inc.

CHAPTER 6 | HORMONE BALANCE

1. Smith, Robyn N, Neil J Mann, Anna Braue, Henna Mäkeläinen, and George A. Varigos. "A Low-Glycemic-Load Diet Improves Symptoms In Acne Vulgaris Patients: A Randomized Controlled Trial". *The American Journal Of Clinical Nutrition* 86, no. 1 (2007): 107-115. doi:10.1093/ajcn/86.1.107

2. Desbonnet, Lieve, Gerard Clarke, Orla O'Sullivan, Paul D. Cotter, Timothy G. Dinan, and John F. Cryan. "Re: Gut Microbiota Depletion From Early Adolescence In Mice: Implications For Brain And Behaviour". *Brain, Behavior, And Immunity* 50 (2015): 335-336. doi:10.1016/j.bbi.2015.07.011.

3. Smith, Robyn N, Neil J Mann, Anna Braue, Henna Mäkeläinen, and George A. Varigos. "A Low-Glycemic-Load Diet Improves Symptoms In Acne Vulgaris Patients: A Randomized Controlled Trial". *The American Journal Of Clinical Nutrition* 86, no. 1 (2007): 107-115. doi:10.1093/ajcn/86.1.107.

4. Chen, Ying, and John Lyga. "Brain-Skin Connection: Stress, Inflammation And Skin Aging". *Inflammation & Allergy-Drug Targets* 13, no. 3 (2014): 177-190. doi:10.2174/1871528113666140522104422.

5. Salem, Iman, Amy Ramser, Nancy Isham, and Mahmoud A. Ghannoum. "The Gut Microbiome As A Major Regulator Of The Gut-Skin Axis". *Frontiers In Microbiology* 9 (2018). doi:10.3389/fmicb.2018.01459.

6. Ellis, Samantha R., Mimi Nguyen, Alexandra R. Vaughn, Manisha Notay, Waqas A. Burney, Simran Sandhu, and Raja K. Sivamani. "The Skin And Gut Microbiome And Its Role In Common Dermatologic Conditions". *Microorganisms* 7, no. 11 (2019): 550. doi:10.3390/microorganisms7110550.

7. Bin Saif, Ghada, Hala Alotaibi, Abdullateef Alzolibani, Noor Almodihesh, Hamad Albraidi, Najed Alotaibi, and Gil Yosipovitch. "Association Of Psychological Stress With Skin Symptoms Among Medical Students". *Saudi Medical Journal* 39, no. 1 (2018): 59-66. doi:10.15537/smj.2018.1.21231.

8. Nagpal, Mohit, Dipankar De, Sanjeev Handa, Arnab Pal, and Naresh Sachdeva. "Insulin Resistance And Metabolic Syndrome In Young Men With Acne". *JAMA Dermatology* 152, no. 4 (2016): 399. doi:10.1001/jamadermatol.2015.4499.

9. O'Neill, Alan M., and Richard L. Gallo. "Host-Microbiome Interactions And Recent Progress Into Understanding The Biology Of Acne Vulgaris". *Microbiome* 6, no. 1 (2018). doi:10.1186/s40168-018-0558-5.

10. "Polycystic Ovary Syndrome PCOS | Endocrine Society". Hormone.Org, 2020. https://www.hormone.org/diseases-and-conditions/polycystic-ovary-syndrome.

11. Yance,Donald R. " *Adaptogens In Medical Herbalism*" (repr., Rochester, Vermont: Healing Arts Press (ITI), 2013), 34-35.

CHAPTER 7 | INFLAMMATION

1. Plewig, Gerd, B Melnik, and WenChieh Chen. *Plewig And Kligman's Acne And Rosacea*, n.d.

2. Burris, MS, RD, Jennifer, William Rietkerk, MD, MBA, and Kathleen Woolf, PhD, RD, FACS. "Acne: The Role Of Medical Nutrition Therapy", 2020. https://jandonline. org/article/S2212-2672(12)01923-5/pdf.

3. P Bowe, W. and Logan C, A., 2011. *Acne Vulgaris, Probiotics And The Gut-Brain-Skin Axis - Back To The Future?*. [online] Gut Pathogens. Available at: <https://gutpathogens.biomedcentral.com/articles/10.1186/1757-4749-3-1> [Accessed 14 October 2019].

4. Smith, R., Mann, N., Braue, A., Mäkeläinen, H. and Varigos, G., 2007. "A low-glycemic-load diet improves symptoms in acne vulgaris patients: a randomized controlled trial". *The American Journal of Clinical Nutrition*, 86(1), pp.107-115.

5. Melnik B. C. (2015). Linking diet to acne metabolomics, inflammation, and comedogenesis: an update. *Clinical, cosmetic and investigational dermatology*, 8, 371–388. https://doi.org/10.2147/CCID.S69135.

6. Lutgendorf, S., Sood, A., Anderson, B., McGinn, S., Maiseri, H., Dao, M., Sorosky, J., De Geest, K., Ritchie, J. and Lubaroff, D., 2005. Social Support, Psychological Distress, and Natural Killer Cell Activity in Ovarian

Cancer. *Journal of Clinical Oncology*, 23(28), pp.7105-7113.

7. Perricone, N., 2003. *Clear Skin Prescription - The Perricone Program To Eliminate Problem Skin*. New York: Harper Collins, pp.9-13.

CHAPTER 8

1. Paterni, I., Granchi, C. and Minutolo, F., 2017. *Risks And Benefits Related To Alimentary Exposure To Xenoestrogens*. [online] Taylor & Francis. Available at: <https://www.tandfonline.com/doi/full/10.1080/10408398.2015.1126547> [Accessed 14 July 2020].

2. EWG. 2020. *Dirty Dozen Endocrine Disruptors*. [online] Available at: <https://www.ewg.org/research/dirty-dozen-list-endocrine-disruptors> [Accessed 14 July 2020].

3. Cdc.gov. 2020. *Dichlorodiphenyltrichloroethane (DDT) Factsheet | National Biomonitoring Program | CDC*. [online] Available at: <https://www.cdc.gov/biomonitoring/DDT_FactSheet.html> [Accessed 14 July 2020].

4. US EPA. 2020. *Persistent Organic Pollutants: A Global Issue, A Global Response | US EPA*. [online] Available at: <https://www.epa.gov/international-cooperation/persistent-organic-pollutants-global-issue-global-response#affect> [Accessed 15 July 2020].

5. NRDC. 2020. *9 Ways To Avoid Hormone-Disrupting Chemicals*. [online] Available at: <https://www.nrdc.org/stories/9-ways-avoid-hormone-disrupting-chemicals> [Accessed 15 July 2020].

6. GBD 2016 Alcohol and Drug Use Collaborators. The global burden of disease attributable to alcohol and drug use in 195 countries and territories, 1990-2016: a systematic analysis for the Global Burden of Disease Study 2016 [published correction appears in Lancet Psychiatry. 2019 Jan;6(1):e2]. *Lancet Psychiatry*. 2018;5(12):987-1012. doi:10.1016/S2215-0366(18)30337-7

7. 10. Mishra VN. Xenoestrogens: The Curse of Civilization. Medicine Update, 2013; 23: 1e.

8. Haelle, T., 2020. *What The Research Says About 10 Controversial Cosmetics Ingredients*. [online] SELF. Available at: <https://www.self.com/story/controversial-cosmetics-ingredients-research> [Accessed 21 July 2020].

9. EWG. 2020. *The Toxic Twelve Chemicals And Contaminants In Cosmetics*. [online] Available at: <https://www.ewg.org/californiacosmetics/toxic12> [Accessed 21 July 2020].

10. EWG. 2020. *Generally Recognized As Safe – But Is It?*. [online] Available at: <https://www.ewg.org/research/ewg-s-dirty-dozen-guide-food-additives/generally-recognized-as-s afe-but-is-it#butylated-hydroxyanisole> [Accessed 21 July 2020].

11. EWG. 2020. *»Bisphenol A*. [online] Available at: <https://www.ewg.org/research/down-drain/%C2%BB-bisphenol> [Accessed 21 July 2020].

12. EWG. 2020. *CVS Will Remove Harmful Ingredients From Sunscreens*. [online] Available at: <https://www.ewg.org/news-and-analysis/2019/08/cvs-will-remove-harmful-ingredients-sunscreen s> [Accessed 21 July 2020].

13. EWG. 2020. *Ask EWG: Lead In Lipstick?*. [online] Available at: <https://www.ewg.org/enviroblog/2007/03/ask-ewg-lead-lipstick> [Accessed 21 July 2020].

14. EWG. 2020. *What Are Parabens, And Why Don'T They Belong In Cosmetics?*. [online] Available at: <https://www.ewg.org/californiacosmetics/parabens> [Accessed 21 July 2020].

15. EWG. 2020. *Dioxin*. [online] Available at: <https://www.ewg.org/release/dioxin/home> [Accessed 21 July 2020].

16. EWG. 2020. *EWG'S Consumer Guide To Seafood*. [online] Available at: <https://www.ewg.org/research/ewgs-good-seafood-guide> [Accessed 21 July 2020].

17. EWG. 2020. *Sample Analysis*. [online] Available at: <https://www.ewg.org/research/pesticides-baby-food/sample-analysis>[Accessed 21 July 2020].

18. EWG. 2020. "What Are Parabens, And Why Don'T They Belong In Cosmetics?".https://www.ewg.org/californiacosmetics/parabens.

19. EWG, 2020. *"BPA And Other Cord Blood Pollutants"*. https://www.ewg.org/research/minority-cord-blood-report/bpa-and-other-cord-blood-pollutants.

20. Formuzis, Alex. *"More Oversight Needed For Cosmetics Made With Talc"*. EWG, 2020. https://www.ewg.org/release/more-oversight-needed-cosmetics-made-talc.

21. Faber, Scott. *"It'S Time To End The Use Of Talc In Loose Powders"*. EWG, 2020. https://www.ewg.org/news-and-analysis/2020/05/it-s-time-end-use-talc-loose-powders.

ACKNOWLEDGEMENTS

Many people have played a role in this book coming to fruition. I want to thank my parents and my brother Terence for their unwavering support and encouragement and for always being willing to be a sounding board. A special thanks to Sheena Liao and Erin Brookins for putting in many hours of hard work throughout this process and always being willing to go the extra mile.

Thank you to my amazing publishing team of Lisa Howard, Editor, Haresh Makwana, Cover Designer, and George Stevens, Interior Designer for taking my vision and bringing it to life while being such a pleasure to work with.

I'd also like to thank Dr. Peter Osborne for helping to connect me with the resources to make this happen and Dr. Matthew Loop for your guidance and support throughout the process and helping me to believe that I could write a best-selling book. Special thanks to Dr. Amit Pandya for being an amazing mentor in dermatology and clinical research.

And thanks also to the doctors who have come before me and who I have been able to learn from across specialties: dermatologists, internists, family practitioners, functional medicine doctors, naturopathic doctors, chiropractors and others. There are too many people to name.

And thanks to my friends and colleagues and also to my subscribers and my social media community! Your excitement and engagement throughout this process has meant the world to me.

RESOURCES

BONUS MATERIALS

To access bonus materials visit ItsNotJustAcne.com/launch-bonuses

RECIPES

Resources for recipes & meal planning adaptable to special diets, organic grass-fed meat, wild caught seafood.
WellAheadChicago.com/resources

SUSTAINABLE SEAFOOD

Get access to a downloadable pocket shopping guide to the best seafood choices based on the state you live in.
Seafoodwatch.org

WATER QUALITY

Information on choosing the best water filter for you
ewg.org/tapwater/water-filter-guide.php
WellAheadChicago.com/resources

ENVIRONMENTAL WORKING GROUP'S SKIN DEEP

This database gives safety ratings for beauty and personal care products, including ratings for individual chemicals that are found in personal care products as well as ratings for products from many popular brands.
www.ewg.org/skindeep

ENVIRONMENTAL WORKING GROUP DIRTY DOZEN

ewg.org/dirty-dozen

MEDICAL GRADE NATURAL SKIN CARE

WellAheadChicago.com/skincare

MEDICAL GRADE SUPPLEMENTS

WellAheadChicago.com/supplements

SPECIALTY LABORATORY TESTING

WellAheadChicago.com/lab-testing

FOOD SOURCES OF NUTRIENTS

The National Institute of Health (NIH) publishes fact sheets on every major vitamin and mineral.
https://ods.od.nih.gov/factsheets/list-VitaminsMinerals

Omega-3s Fatty Acids
- Wild-caught seafood (i.e., sardines, salmon, cod, shrimp, crab, etc.)
- Grass-fed beef

Omega-9 Fatty Acids
- Olive oil
- Avocados
- Almonds
- Almond oil
- High-oleic safflower oil

Zinc

- → Oysters
- → Red meat
- → Poultry
- → Beans
- → Cashews
- → Almonds

Vitamin A

- → Egg yolks
- → Beef liver
- → Butter
- → Salmon
- → Cod liver oil
- → Chicken liver

Vitamin B6

- → Banana
- → Avocado
- → Sweet potato with the skin
- → Potatoes with the skin
- → Organ meats
- → Salmon
- → Chicken breast
- → Turkey breast
- → Sunflower seeds

Vitamin D

- → Sockeye salmon
- → Trout
- → Cod liver oil
- → Dried mushrooms

Vitamin E

- ➜ Sunflower oil
- ➜ Sunflower seeds
- ➜ Almonds
- ➜ Hazelnuts- Avocados
- ➜ Dark leafy greens
- ➜ Butternut squash
- ➜ Kiwi fruit

Selenium

- ➜ Brazil nuts, mixed nuts
- ➜ Whole eggs, cooked
- ➜ Oysters
- ➜ Fish
- ➜ Organ meats - Red meat
- ➜ Poultry

Niacin

- ➜ Mushrooms
- ➜ Potatoes
- ➜ Organ meats

Biotin

- ➜ Beef liver
- ➜ Legumes
- ➜ Whole eggs, cooked
- ➜ Fish
- ➜ Pork

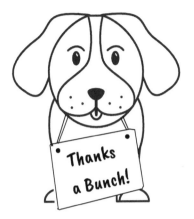

I really appreciate all of your support and I love hearing what you have to say.

I'm so excited for you to get started on this journey towards clear skin and total health. I can't wait to hear how It's Not Just Acne is changing your life!

Help another reader know if this book is for them by leaving a review on Amazon. Thanks so much!!

bit.ly/acnebookreview

Made in the USA
Columbia, SC
14 December 2023

28547215R00083